The Human Side of Medical Training

When Things Don't Go as Planned

How to Make Sense of Setbacks, Remediation, and What Comes Next in Medical School

Laura S. Woodward, Ph.D.

THRESHOLD ACADEMIC PRESS
Royal Oak, Michigan

This book is intended for educational purposes only. It does not provide medical or mental health care and is not a substitute for professional care, academic advising, clinical supervision, or institutional guidance. The frameworks and examples presented here are intended to support thinking about learning and performance under pressure, not to diagnose or treat distress.

Readers experiencing persistent or worsening distress, illness, substantial difficulty functioning, concerns about safety, or academic difficulties beyond the scope of this book should seek support appropriate to the situation from qualified professionals, supervisors, advisors, or institutional resources.

The information in this book reflects the author's interpretation of research and educational practice at the time of writing. Research findings, educational practices, and institutional policies may change over time.

Artificial intelligence tools were used to assist in the preparation of this book, under the author's direction, editing, and final review. The author is responsible for the final content.

First edition.

ISBN: 979-8-9978928-0-7

Library of Congress Control Number: 2026923112

Printed in the United States of America

thresholdacademicpress@gmail.com

Contents

Start with What Is Happening

After a setback, most readers do not need a perfect reading plan. They need the next section that matches the problem in front of them.

Use the book by the question you are carrying today:

You do not need to know where you belong in the whole book. Start with the closest match.

If this is where you are	Start here
Something just happened, and the meaning is expanding quickly.	Introduction and Part I
You need to understand where the problem actually lives.	Part II
You know something needs to change, but you are having trouble functioning enough to act.	Part III
The formal decision has happened, and now you are dealing with loss, timeline change, return, or identity.	Part IV
You are advising, supervising, or supporting a learner.	After Ch. 11, and Notes for Educators

Read enough to locate the problem more accurately. Then choose one next action and stop before the book becomes one more thing to complete.

When More Support Would Help

A book can help you name what is happening, lower the noise around it, and decide what to ask next. It cannot replace clinical care, urgent support, supervision, advising, or someone who can stay with you when safety is in question.

Please reach for more support now if you are thinking about suicide, feeling at risk of hurting yourself or someone else, unable to stay safe, or unsure you can make it through the next stretch without immediate help. Please reach for more support soon if distress is worsening, functioning is dropping, sleep or eating has changed enough to affect daily life, substances are becoming part of how you get through the day, or people close to you are worried about your safety.

In the United States, you can call or text 988 or use 988 Lifeline chat. In Canada, you can call or text 988. In any location, use the local emergency number or go to the nearest emergency department if there is immediate danger.

Within a training program, support may also include your physician or clinician, campus counseling, employee assistance, disability or accommodation services, the dean of students, the GME office, your program director, a chief resident, a trusted supervisor, or a local crisis team. You do not need to decide which category your distress belongs in before reaching for a real person.

Getting support is not evidence that the setback is larger than you thought. It is one way to stop carrying it alone.

Introduction: Medical Education Teaches Success Better Than Recovery

After a failed exam or difficult evaluation, the first problem is usually concrete. You need to find out what happens next, who you need to contact, and whether there is a deadline. The other questions tend to arrive before those answers do.

- *What does this mean about me?*
- *Was I never as capable as I thought?*
- *Does everyone know?*
- *Do I still belong here?*
- *Have I ruined my future?*

Medical training prepares you well for forward motion. There is always another course, another rotation, another exam, another application, another level of responsibility.

The sequence is visible. You know where you are supposed to be and what is supposed to happen next. When that sequence breaks, the practical problem can quickly become a much larger one.

You fail an exam by three points. Twenty minutes later, you are searching for what remediation might mean for residency. You receive one difficult evaluation and begin wondering whether every supervisor has been thinking the same thing. By the next morning, you may know far more about the worst possible outcome than you know about what actually went wrong.

When you do not yet know what the result means, your mind starts filling in the missing pieces. That is often when a failed exam becomes a prediction about residency, or one evaluation starts to feel like a verdict on your ability.

A program can tell you that you failed an exam. That does not tell you why you failed it.

A supervisor can tell you that your clinical reasoning was below expectations. That does not tell you whether the concern appears across settings, whether other supervisors have seen the same thing, or exactly what needs to improve.

Remediation tells you that more work is required. It does not tell you that you were never capable of becoming a physician.

Sometimes the problem turns out to be fairly clear. You did not know enough. You prepared in a way that did not match the task. You missed feedback you needed to take seriously.

Other situations are harder to untangle. You may have been exhausted, sick, overloaded, poorly supervised, unclear about what was expected, or dealing with something outside training. Several of those things can be present at the same time, and the outcome alone cannot tell you which mattered most.

This book starts before that larger judgment gets made. Sometimes the investigation will uncover a real weakness, a pattern that needs correction, or a consequence you cannot avoid.

The work is to find out what actually requires attention before turning one event into a conclusion about your ability, character, or future. The sequence is simple:

Event before conclusion. Locate before you label. Diagnose before you redesign.

Start with what happened. If you failed an exam, begin with the exam. What did the score report show? Where were the gaps? What was happening during the period when you prepared? What information are you still missing?

If a supervisor raised a concern, get specific. What did they observe? Was the feedback about knowledge, reasoning, communication, efficiency, professionalism, or something else? Has anyone else raised the same concern?

If training has been interrupted, find out what has actually changed. What is required now? What remains uncertain? Which consequences are established, and which ones are fears about what might happen later?

None of those questions is as immediate as *What does this say about me?* They are still the questions that tell you what to do next.

Medical training can make this difficult because performance is never completely separate from identity. You are being taught, evaluated, supervised, compared with standards, and gradually trusted with more responsibility. A poor result can therefore feel larger than the task that produced it.

The exam can begin to feel like evidence about intelligence. The evaluation can feel like evidence about whether you belong. A delayed timeline can feel like evidence that everyone else is moving forward while you have become someone who fell behind.

Those reactions matter, especially when the setback has disrupted how you understood your place in training. You still do not have to decide immediately what they mean about your future.

You may eventually learn that the problem was narrower than you feared. You may discover that the concern was real and needs substantial work. You may find that the environment contributed in ways that also need to be addressed.

What matters early on is resisting the urge to decide the whole meaning of the event before you understand the event itself. That can be especially hard when uncertainty feels worse than a harsh explanation.

I am not capable is painful, but it is complete. *I do not yet know why this happened* leaves the question open — and the open question is often the more accurate one.

Early on, you usually do not have enough information to decide what the setback means for your future. For now, there are smaller questions to answer. What happened? What evidence do you have? What are you assuming? What needs attention first?

Start there. The rest can wait until there is enough information to know what it deserves to mean.

Part I: When Something Goes Wrong

A setback can become bigger in your mind before you have had time to understand it. You fail an exam and start thinking about residency. You receive one difficult evaluation and wonder whether everyone has been thinking the same thing. You are told to remediate and begin reconsidering years of evidence about your ability.

The event is real. The conclusions that follow may be moving faster than the information. Part I starts with a narrower question:

What happened, and what does it not yet tell me?

That question does not minimize the problem. It gives you somewhere accurate to begin.

Chapter 1: Setbacks Are Part of the Training Landscape

You open the score report and see the number first. Sixty-two percent, with sixty-five required to pass. You check it again, then look for the class average or topic breakdown, hoping some detail will make the result easier to understand. Within minutes, your attention has moved far beyond the exam. *Maybe I have finally reached my limit.*

That thought can carry unusual force for someone who has spent years succeeding. You worked hard, performed well, and learned that effort usually led to progress. Medical training reinforced the pattern as one course led to another, then to rotations, applications, and greater responsibility. Success gradually became part of the evidence that you belonged. A major interruption can suddenly make competence, belonging, and the imagined future feel less certain. Medical students interviewed after assessment failure and remediation have described strong shame, self-doubt, and concerns about what the event meant for their suitability and future in medicine (Mills et al., 2024).

Most of what you see around you supports the story of smooth progress. Classmates begin the next block, residents move up a year, and people match, graduate, publish, and take on new roles. You see much less of the repeated exams, difficult evaluations, informal coaching, leaves, and remediation plans that usually remain private. Some trainees do move through long stretches of training without major disruption. What you can see is mostly the part of training that moved forward.

You know your own record in a way you will never know most other people's. You remember the exam you barely passed, the material that took longer than expected, and the feedback you still think about months later. You also know about the week you could not concentrate or the period when you were functioning below your usual level. Much of that information disappears when you look at another student or resident from the outside. You are comparing your complete record with everyone else's public record.

That comparison can make one setback feel unusually revealing. Research on struggling learners describes heterogeneous difficulties involving knowledge, clinical skills, professionalism, personal circumstances, and combinations of these problems (Lacasse et al., 2019; Montreuil et al., 2025). More recent reviews also show that the field does not consistently define either the struggling learner or remediation itself (Percival et al., 2026). There is no single profile that explains every trainee who runs into difficulty. There is also no reason to pretend that everyone struggles in the same way. What you can see around you tells you less than it appears to.

A setback may also expose assumptions you did not know you were carrying. You may have believed that competent students do not fail exams, strong residents do not need remediation, or capable people recover quickly when something goes wrong. Those beliefs are rarely stated directly, yet they can become part of how you measure yourself. Professional identity develops through participation, evaluation, relationships, and the process of becoming recognized as a physician (Monrouxe, 2010). Performance can therefore begin to feel like information about who you are becoming.

A Setback Can Matter Without Explaining Everything

A setback deserves attention because something happened that did not go as expected. A failed examination may reveal a knowledge gap, a study approach that did not work well enough, or difficulty using knowledge under testing conditions. Illness, exhaustion, competing responsibilities, or several problems together may also have affected the result. A concerning clinical evaluation may raise questions about reasoning, communication, procedural skill, efficiency, professionalism, supervision, or expectations. The outcome gives you a reason to investigate, not an explanation by itself.

Two responses can interfere with that investigation. You can decide immediately that the setback proves something fundamental about you, or you can dismiss it with phrases such as *everyone struggles* and *failure is part of the process*. The first response makes the conclusion too large too quickly. The second can make a meaningful problem seem smaller than it is. Neither tells you what needs attention.

It can help to know that difficulty in training is not unusual, especially if that knowledge makes it easier to look closely at your own situation. A repeated concern still matters, and a real deficit still requires correction. **Normalization should reduce shame without reducing curiosity.**

Why Medicine Makes a Setback Feel So Personal

A poor result in medical training rarely stays confined to the task itself. The people teaching you may also evaluate you, and the institution helping you develop may also decide whether you progress. A supervisor can be teacher, mentor, assessor, and gatekeeper within the same period of training. Performance information therefore carries social and professional weight alongside its educational meaning. A narrow problem can begin to feel like a judgment about your place in medicine.

The questions often widen quickly. *How did I perform?* becomes *How am I being seen?* A remediation plan may make you wonder whether faculty now think differently about you or whether your classmates know. A scoping review of medical students experiencing academic difficulty identified themes of identity preservation and apprehension toward the medical school's dual role as both a source of support and a gatekeeper to progression (Kirtchuk et al., 2022). The very system you may need for support can also feel like the system you need to protect yourself from.

The learning environment belongs in the picture as well. Research has linked characteristics of the medical-school learning environment with outcomes including exhaustion and career regret, although those findings cannot explain why a particular learner failed an exam or received difficult feedback (Dyrbye et al., 2021). A resident may need to improve prioritization while also learning an unfamiliar workflow under inconsistent supervision. A student may need a better study approach while also dealing with illness, caregiving, or severe disruption outside school. A learner brings knowledge, skill, health, preparation, and judgment into an assessment. The assessment also happens inside a workload, a supervisory structure, and a set of expectations.

Labels Feel Clearer Than They Are

Labels become attractive when you want uncertainty to end. Words such as *lazy*, *weak*, *disorganized*, *unprofessional*, or *not smart enough* sound complete because they are short and definite. They can hide several different problems under the same description. Once the label takes over, it becomes harder to see what actually needs to change. Removing the label usually produces better questions.

Suppose a resident is told that they are too slow. The resident may have trouble prioritizing, spend too long documenting, lack enough knowledge to make decisions efficiently, or repeatedly check work because they are afraid of missing something. The workflow may also be unfamiliar, the service may be overloaded, or different supervisors may expect different things. Several explanations could be operating at the same time. The word *slow* tells you where the problem became visible, not where it began.

The same thing happens when learners label themselves. *I failed because I am lazy* sounds explanatory until you ask what the word describes. Did you study less than you planned, avoid the hardest material, rely heavily on passive review, or struggle to use the time you had? Were you also exhausted, ill, distracted, or carrying responsibilities that changed what you could realistically do? The answers may still be uncomfortable. At least they tell you what actually needs attention.

Start With What You Know

The first useful move is to separate the event from the conclusions already gathering around it. A score of sixty-two percent when sixty-five was required to pass is a fact. *I cannot handle medical school* is an interpretation of that fact. The interpretation may express a real fear, but the score alone cannot establish it. Keeping those statements separate gives you somewhere concrete to begin.

The Fact/Inference Split

You do not need to complete this carefully or completely. A few phrases are enough to begin.

Divide a page into two columns.

What I know

- My score was 62 percent.
- Passing was 65 percent.
- My weakest areas were renal and cardiovascular.
- I slept about four hours the night before.
- I have been asked to meet with the course director.

What I am inferring

- I cannot handle medical school.
- Everyone else understood the material.

- Faculty will think I do not belong here.
- This will ruin residency.
- I will probably fail again.

The second column may contain concerns worth taking seriously. Some may become more plausible as you gather information. The exercise does not ask you to argue with them or replace them with reassuring thoughts. It asks you to notice that they require evidence the first column does not provide. That distinction keeps the event from answering questions that are still open.

The two columns can blur quickly after something goes wrong. *I failed this exam* can become *I am failing at medicine,* and *one supervisor raised a concern* can become *everyone thinks I am weak. I have to remediate* can become *my future is ruined* before the consequences are even clear. The first statement in each pair gives you something to investigate. The second asks the event to explain more than you currently know.

A setback can be painful, consequential, and important. It may reveal something that genuinely needs to change. It can also grow in meaning before enough information exists to explain it. The first task is to resist that expansion long enough to see what the event actually shows. **A setback deserves investigation before interpretation.**

Chapter 2: The Event Is Not the Whole Story

A resident finishes a rotation and opens the evaluation portal at home. Most of the comments are familiar, and then one sentence stops her: *Clinical reasoning below expectations for level of training.* She reads it again, then begins wondering whether other supervisors have thought the same thing. Within minutes, one evaluation has raised questions about competence, reputation, and the future. The words on the screen are specific, but their meaning is already expanding.

What Happened, and What Did It Touch?

A performance problem can affect more than the skill being evaluated. The resident may wonder whether she can reason well enough to care for patients, whether the attending now sees her differently, and whether she still belongs at this level of training. She may also begin questioning assumptions that felt stable the day before. A future that seemed predictable can suddenly feel uncertain. One event can therefore disturb several parts of how a learner understands themselves and their place in medicine.

That widening can happen before the original event has been examined closely. The attending may have observed a real problem, but the resident may not yet know what behavior led to the rating. She may not know whether the concern appeared throughout the rotation or during a few difficult cases. She may have no idea whether other supervisors have seen the same pattern. The feeling that everything has changed can arrive long before the evidence shows how much has actually changed.

This distinction is useful because the event and its impact are different kinds of information. The event might be one failed examination, one concerning evaluation, or one requirement to remediate. What it touches may include competence, belonging, expectations, professional identity, and plans for the future. Those reactions are real even when the larger conclusions remain uncertain. Understanding what was shaken does not require assuming that everything it touched has been lost.

Keep the Claim as Narrow as the Evidence

Evaluation matters in medicine because trainees are gradually being trusted with greater responsibility. Professional identity also develops through participation, recognition, and the social process of becoming a physician (Monrouxe, 2010). Feedback can therefore land in a place that already carries a great deal of personal meaning. A learner may hear information about a particular behavior and experience it as information about the kind of physician they are becoming. That is one reason specificity matters so much.

Suppose a resident is told that her handoffs are incomplete. A more useful description would identify what is missing, such as pending tests, contingency plans, or changes that occurred late in the shift. Now the resident has a behavior that can be observed and corrected. A conclusion such as *I am an unsafe doctor* stretches the information far beyond what was actually described. Once the claim becomes specific enough to observe, the learner can start checking whether it is accurate and what would need to change.

The same process applies to clinical reasoning. *I am bad at clinical reasoning* covers too much territory to guide improvement. *One attending said I had trouble prioritizing the differential during oral presentations* is narrower and gives the learner something to investigate. The next questions become practical: Did other supervisors see this, did it occur in other settings, and what specifically happened during the presentations? A smaller claim can produce a more serious and useful investigation.

Precision does not protect the learner from difficult evidence. A repeated problem with handoffs may be important, and a consistent weakness in clinical reasoning may require substantial work. The advantage of specificity is that it keeps the problem attached to what can actually be examined. Broad judgments often feel more severe while giving the learner less direction. Specific information tells the learner what they are actually being asked to improve.

When a Performance Problem Becomes a Judgment About the Self

After a setback, criticism can shift from something you did to something you believe you are. *I prepared poorly for this exam* can become *I am lazy*, and *I missed important findings* can become *I should not be trusted with patients*. The first statements describe actions or performance that can be examined. The second statements make the entire person the problem. That change may happen so quickly that the learner barely notices it.

Research on shame in medical learners describes experiences involving global negative self-evaluation, threats to self-concept, and questions about whether the learner belongs in medicine (Bynum et al., 2019; Bynum et al., 2021a; Bynum et al., 2021b). Work on shame and guilt also distinguishes between criticism directed toward an action and criticism directed toward the self more broadly, a distinction that has also been applied specifically to how medical learners respond to their own errors (Tangney & Dearing, 2002; Bynum & Goodie, 2014). Those distinctions can help explain why some feedback feels much larger than the behavior being discussed. They do not mean that every setback produces shame. Learners may also feel disappointment, anger, anxiety, embarrassment, confusion, defensiveness, relief, or very little emotional disruption.

The useful question is where the criticism has landed. *I underestimated how much practice I needed* gives you a behavior to examine. *I am someone who does not work hard enough* turns one problem into a description of character. A harsher judgment can feel more honest, especially when you are disappointed in yourself. It still tells you less about what happened and what needs to change.

Specificity becomes especially important when the concern is genuinely yours. If you arrived late three times and failed to notify the team twice, those behaviors need attention. Calling yourself irresponsible does not add much information about why it happened or what needs to change. You may eventually discover a pattern that deserves serious correction. The work begins by describing the pattern accurately.

When One Event Starts Explaining the Past

A setback can change the way earlier experiences look. After one failed exam, the anatomy course that felt difficult two years ago may suddenly seem significant. A comment about being more concise can start to look like early evidence of a larger clinical problem. Experiences that once seemed separate begin lining up into a single story. The present event starts reorganizing the past.

This can be especially powerful when the setback conflicts with the person you expected yourself to be. Higgins's self-discrepancy theory describes distress that can arise when actual experience differs from important expectations about the self (Higgins, 1987). This theoretical approach helps explain why a learner who expected to be someone who succeeds may experience a major disruption when that expectation is challenged. The event creates uncertainty about more than the immediate task. The learner begins looking for an explanation that makes the new experience fit.

One possible sequence looks like this. The event is *I failed the exam,* and the disruption is *I thought my preparation was working.* The explanation becomes *maybe I understand less than I thought,* and the larger conclusion becomes *I am not capable of succeeding here.* Each step moves farther from what the score alone establishes. This sequence is used throughout this book, though it resonates with recent theoretical work describing how uncertainty about a professional situation can become personalized into uncertainty about one's own worth, which can in turn resolve into a felt certainty about lacking that worth (Han et al., 2026). It is not a single established psychological mechanism confirmed for every training setback.

A large conclusion can be strangely appealing because it ends the uncertainty. *I am not capable* is painful, but it feels complete. *I do not yet understand why this happened* leaves uncertainty in place. Medical training gives learners many reasons to dislike uncertainty when progression and future opportunities may be involved. A complete explanation can therefore feel convincing before it is well supported.

Make the Problem Smaller Before You Make It Bigger

A broad statement becomes more useful when you keep narrowing it. Start with *I am bad at clinical reasoning,* then move to *my clinical reasoning was rated poorly on this rotation.* Narrow it again to *one attending rated my reasoning below expectations.* Then identify what the attending actually observed, such as difficulty prioritizing the differential during oral presentations. At that point, you finally have something that can be checked.

The next question is whether the pattern appears elsewhere. Previous evaluations may show similar concerns, or they may show consistently strong performance. Other supervisors may have observed the same problem, or the concern may be limited to one setting. Direct observation may clarify whether the difficulty lies in reasoning itself or in communicating the reasoning clearly. Evidence can make the concern more serious, less serious, or simply more specific.

Narrowing a problem is sometimes mistaken for minimizing it. The opposite can happen when specificity reveals a pattern that broad language had hidden. Three supervisors independently identifying the same behavior deserves more attention than one vague comment. A repeated problem across settings may require substantial correction. Once the problem is described accurately, you can decide whether it needs a small adjustment, sustained remediation, or more information before either response makes sense.

What the Event Does Not Yet Tell You

An event can establish something important without answering every question that follows. A failed exam establishes that the passing standard was not met on that assessment. A concerning evaluation establishes that an evaluator identified a problem under particular circumstances. A remediation decision establishes that additional work is required. None of those facts automatically explains the cause, scope, duration, or future consequence of the problem.

Several questions remain open until more evidence is available. Does the concern appear across settings, or was it limited to one context? Did multiple observers identify the same behavior, and were they in a position to see it clearly? Were expectations known, and does contradictory evidence exist elsewhere in the learner's record? These questions determine how much weight the event deserves.

Event → Disruption → Explanation → Conclusion

Take one setback and write a brief answer to each prompt.

Event

What happened that another person could reasonably verify?

Disruption

What expectation, plan, assumption, or sense of competence did the event disturb?

Explanation

What do you currently think caused the problem?

Conclusion

What larger claim have you started making about yourself, your belonging, or your future?

Evidence needed

What would you need to know before that conclusion was justified?

A completed example might begin with one attending rating clinical reasoning below expectations. The disruption might be that the learner believed the rotation was going well, while the current explanation is difficulty prioritizing the differential during presentations. The larger conclusion might be *I am going to be a poor physician*. Useful evidence would include examples from the evaluator, observations from other supervisors, previous evaluations, and performance in other settings. The exercise helps separate what is established from what still needs investigation.

Some concerns will become stronger after that investigation. If several supervisors independently describe the same behavior across different settings, the learner has more reason to treat the pattern seriously. If the concern disappears when the behavior is observed directly, the explanation may need revision. The purpose is not to make every conclusion less threatening. The purpose is to make it answerable to evidence.

A real problem may require substantial correction. It can affect progression, require remediation, or expose a pattern that the learner needs to address. Those consequences do not make every conclusion drawn from the event accurate. The first responsibility is to understand how far the evidence actually reaches. A problem becomes more workable when its description stays close to what is known.

Chapter 3: Why Thinking Gets Harder After a Setback

The morning after a failed exam, you may know exactly what you need to do. You need to open the score report, contact the course director, review the weak areas, and find out what happens next. Two hours later, you have reread the same email six times, searched residency forums, opened the study platform, and closed it again. Then a second problem appears: *Why can't I even deal with this properly?* The difficulty responding starts to feel like more evidence that something is wrong.

That conclusion can arrive too quickly. A setback changes more than your schedule because familiar tasks can suddenly carry consequences, uncertainty, and fear about what they might reveal. Reading the score report is no longer just reading a score report, and meeting with a supervisor is no longer just a meeting. You may be trying to solve several problems at the same time before you have enough information to solve any of them well. Before deciding that your concentration has failed, look at what your attention is being asked to carry.

Too Many Things Are Asking for Your Attention

Working memory and attentional control are limited, and anxiety or acute stress can reduce processing efficiency when demanding tasks require attention, working memory, retrieval, or decision-making (Eysenck et al., 2007; LeBlanc, 2009). After a setback, you may be studying while also replaying what happened, predicting future consequences, monitoring your concentration, and wondering how other people see you. Each of those demands takes up some of the same limited attention you need for the work itself.

This is a functional explanation, not a diagnosis of why any particular learner is struggling. Poor sleep, illness, anxiety, depression, medication effects, life disruption, and many other factors can affect concentration and functioning. The evidence cited here supports the narrower point that limited cognitive capacity and competing attention can make demanding tasks harder. It does not establish that every learner who feels scattered after a setback is experiencing the same mechanism. Persistent or substantial difficulty functioning deserves attention on its own terms.

When Thinking Stops Producing Anything New

Thinking about a setback is often necessary. You may need to review what happened, understand feedback, decide whether to appeal, or work out what to say in an upcoming meeting. Repetitive thought is not uniformly helpful or harmful; its effects depend partly on how the thinking is conducted and what it produces (Watkins, 2008). In practical terms, useful analysis tends to generate new information, a decision, another question, or a next action, while unproductive repetition can return you to the same unanswered question without changing what you know.

Consider the question *Why did I fail?* Reviewing the score breakdown, comparing it with how you prepared, and identifying weak domains can give you new information. Asking yourself for the fiftieth time how you could have allowed this to happen may leave you with exactly what you knew before. The thought feels urgent because the setback matters, but urgency does not make the question answerable through repetition. One way to tell the difference is to ask what the thinking has produced. Do you know something new, have a decision to make, or know what you need to do next?

The point is not to stop thinking about what happened. Some problems require careful thought, and difficult information may need to be revisited more than once. The problem begins when you keep asking incomplete information to provide certainty it cannot. At that point, more thinking may feel like work without moving the problem forward. That distinction can help you decide whether you need more analysis or new information.

When Studying Becomes Another Examination

After a setback, ordinary practice can start feeling like a test of whether you have recovered. You miss one question and think, *See, I still don't understand this.* You reread the same paragraph twice and decide your concentration is gone. You feel anxious before a presentation and take the anxiety itself as evidence that you are not ready. Now you are doing the work while also grading what the work supposedly says about you.

Medical learners do not simply receive performance information and accept it at face value. They make judgments about its credibility, meaning, and relevance to themselves (Watling et al., 2012). After a threatening setback, ordinary cues during practice may begin to feel like evidence about future competence. One missed question can become proof that the new study plan is failing, and one awkward presentation can become proof that you returned too soon. Practice becomes much harder to interpret when every moment is treated as a final assessment.

This matters because practice normally contains mistakes. Studying includes imperfect recall, uneven concentration, confusion, and questions you cannot answer on the first attempt. Clinical learning also includes hesitations, correction, and feedback because those are part of learning the work. If every error becomes evidence about whether you still belong, practice stops functioning as practice. You need room to do the work without turning each attempt into a conclusion about the whole recovery process.

Why Avoidance Can Start Here

A task can become harder to approach after its meaning changes. Before the failed exam, opening the question bank may have meant *I am going to study for an hour*. Afterward, it may mean *I am about to find out whether I can still do this*. Before the difficult evaluation, meeting with the course director may have meant *I need information*. Now it may feel like walking into a room where someone is about to explain what your future looks like.

That change in meaning can contribute to avoidance. The score report stays unopened, the email remains a draft, or you study everything except the material that caused trouble. From the outside, this may look like procrastination or poor follow-through. Sometimes that description is accurate, and avoidance can have many causes. Other times, the learner is struggling to approach what the task has come to represent.

The distinction matters because difficulty beginning is not automatic evidence that your capacity has disappeared. The task may now carry fear, embarrassment, or uncertainty that was absent before the setback. This does not remove the need to respond, especially when deadlines or consequences are involved. It does help explain why telling yourself to *just do it* may fail when the task has become emotionally loaded. Chapter 7 returns to avoidance in more detail once the underlying problem has been investigated.

Emotional Urgency Is Different From Actual Urgency

A setback can make almost every question feel as though it needs an answer immediately. Some questions truly are time-sensitive because an appeal deadline, required meeting, patient-safety issue, accommodation request, or administrative response cannot wait. Those items deserve priority because delay changes what happens next. Other questions feel just as urgent while remaining impossible to answer with the information currently available. The feeling of urgency and the presence of a deadline are different things.

Questions such as *Does this prove I am not capable?* or *Will everyone see me differently now?* may demand attention all night. You can spend hours trying to settle whether the setback will follow you forever or has ruined the career you imagined. The problem is that these questions often depend on information that does not exist yet. Thinking harder cannot supply an evaluation that has not been written, a policy you have not read, or evidence about future performance you have not yet produced. Before treating a question as urgent, check whether delay would actually change anything.

This distinction does not justify delaying something that genuinely needs action. If an appeal closes tomorrow, the deadline matters even if you feel overwhelmed. If a supervisor needs a response or there is an immediate safety concern, those tasks belong at the front of the line. The distinction keeps urgent tasks from being crowded out by larger questions you cannot yet answer. You do not have to solve your entire future to send the email that is due today.

Sometimes the Problem Is Missing Information

A decision can feel impossible because you do not yet have what you need to make it. Whether to appeal an exam result may depend on the written policy, the deadline, the score breakdown, and the grounds that qualify for review. Whether one evaluation reflects a pattern may require previous evaluations, another supervisor's observations, or clarification from the person who wrote it. More thinking cannot substitute for information that has not been gathered. If the missing piece is a policy, deadline, score report, or supervisor's observation, more reflection will not supply it. The next move is to get the information.

This is an important distinction after a setback because confusion can easily be mistaken for incapacity. You may sit for an hour trying to decide what to do when the decision cannot yet be made responsibly. The useful question becomes: **Am I unable to decide because I cannot think clearly, or because I do not yet have the information required to decide?** Those are different problems and call for different next steps. One may require reducing cognitive load, while the other requires finding the missing fact.

Cognitive Triage

When several problems feel urgent at once, sorting them is often more useful than trying to solve them all. The point of triage is to identify which questions require action, which require information, and which can remain unanswered for now. It should take only a few minutes and does not require you to feel calm before you begin. A page is enough. Use the categories below to decide what deserves your attention first.

What requires action now?

List only items with a real reason they cannot wait, such as a deadline, required email, confirmed meeting, safety concern, or urgent health need.

What information am I missing?

List facts you need before you can make a useful decision, such as the score breakdown, written policy, specific feedback, or remediation requirements.

What am I trying to answer too early?

Name the larger question your mind keeps trying to settle before the necessary evidence exists.

What can remain unanswered for now?

Complete the sentence: *I do not have enough information yet to decide ___________.*

What am I repeatedly thinking about without generating anything new?

Write down the question or thought that keeps returning, then identify whether it points to evidence, a decision, an action, or nothing you can currently resolve.

Triage does not make serious problems disappear. A deadline is still a deadline, a real performance concern still needs attention, and persistent difficulty functioning still deserves appropriate support. What triage can do is stop every concern from competing for first place at the same time. It separates the problem that needs an email today from the question about your future that may take months to answer. That separation can make the next hour more manageable.

The Second Conclusion

A setback can produce one painful conclusion, then use your reaction to support another. The first may be *I am not capable*, while the second becomes *the fact that I cannot handle this properly proves it*. Difficulty concentrating, sleeping, organizing yourself, or approaching the work is then treated as confirmation of the original fear. The reaction to the setback becomes evidence about the cause of the setback. That is a leap worth noticing.

There are many reasons someone may function poorly after difficult news. A learner may be embarrassed, exhausted, distracted, missing information, sleeping badly, or trying to solve too many problems at once. None of those possibilities proves that the original academic or clinical concern was minor. They also do not establish that professional capacity disappeared overnight. **Do not use the difficulty of responding to the setback as automatic proof of what the setback supposedly says about you.**

Persistent difficulty functioning should still be taken seriously. If concentration, sleep, mood, or daily functioning remain substantially impaired, that may require support beyond the educational problem itself. The point here is narrower than saying the reaction will always pass. Your immediate difficulty responding is information about how you are functioning after the event. It is not yet an explanation of why the event happened.

The reaction to a setback can tell you something important about what the learner is carrying afterward. It cannot tell you, by itself, whether the original problem was knowledge, skill, strategy, health, environment, or something else. Part I has deliberately stayed with what happens after the event without pretending that the reaction explains the event itself. The next task is to investigate the problem that produced the outcome. **Event before conclusion. Now, locate before you label.**

Part II: What Actually Went Wrong?

Once the first shock settles, a harder question remains: why did this happen? A failed exam, difficult evaluation, or remediation decision tells you where a problem became visible, but it does not tell you where the problem began. The explanation may lie mainly in the learner, mainly in the environment, or in the way the two interacted. More than one explanation may fit at first. The next task is to sort among them.

That requires a different kind of thinking from the first days after a setback. Start by locating where the problem might live, then consider the explanations that could reasonably account for what happened. After that, test those explanations against the evidence you actually have. Medical-education work on remediation similarly emphasizes identifying the specific difficulty, assessing contributing factors, and matching intervention to the learner's needs, while also acknowledging that the evidence base remains uneven and remediation itself is not uniformly defined (Chou et al., 2019; Montreuil et al., 2025; Percival et al., 2026). The aim is simple: understand the problem well enough that the next action has a reason behind it.

Locate. Differentiate. Test.

The question now is no longer *What does this say about me?* The question is: **What kind of problem is this, where does it live, and what evidence supports that conclusion?**

Chapter 4: Locate Before You Label

When something goes wrong, the learner usually receives the result first. The failed score is yours, the evaluation has your name on it, and the remediation meeting is on your calendar. That makes it easy to assume that the cause must also be located entirely in you. Sometimes that conclusion is right. Sometimes it is only the first explanation available.

The result tells you where the problem became visible. It does not automatically tell you where the problem began. A poor outcome can come mainly from the learner, mainly from the environment, or from the way the two interacted. More than one source may be contributing at the same time. Before deciding what kind of learner problem this is, identify where the difficulty may actually be coming from.

Three Places a Problem Can Live

Some problems are primarily learner problems. A student may have a knowledge gap, a resident may struggle to prioritize, or a trainee may repeatedly ignore feedback that has been clear and specific. Those problems belong to the learner and need direct attention. The surrounding environment may still affect how easy they are to correct. The responsibility for change begins where the problem actually is.

Other problems are primarily environmental. Expectations may be unclear, supervision may be inconsistent, workload may be unreasonable, or the learner may be receiving contradictory guidance from different supervisors. In those situations, asking the learner to simply work harder may leave the central problem untouched. The learner may still need to adapt in the short term. The environment also has something that needs to change.

Many setbacks sit between those two categories. A resident who is slow on rounds may genuinely need to improve prioritization while also working in an unfamiliar system with a heavy patient load and unclear expectations. A student may need a better study method while also trying to learn during illness, caregiving, or severe schedule disruption. The learner and the environment can both contribute to the same outcome. That makes the problem harder to sort out, but it also makes a single label less useful.

What Does "Too Slow" Actually Mean?

Imagine a resident who is repeatedly told they are too slow. That phrase sounds clear until you try to decide what should change. The resident may be spending too long documenting, hesitating because they are unsure what matters most, or working slowly because their knowledge is not yet automatic. They may also be new to the workflow, carrying more patients than usual, or receiving different expectations from different supervisors. The label identifies the complaint without explaining the cause.

The useful question is: **If I removed the label, what behavior would be left?** Instead of *too slow*, you might find that the resident takes twenty minutes to complete notes because they rewrite the assessment several times. Instead of *disorganized*, you might find that a student repeatedly misses deadlines because they are tracking tasks in several places and overlooking messages. Instead of *unprofessional*, you might find that a learner has arrived late three times without notifying the team. Behavior gives you something you can examine.

This matters because labels compress different problems into the same word. Two residents can both be called inefficient while needing completely different interventions. One may need stronger clinical knowledge, while the other needs a better workflow. A third may be functioning adequately in an environment that is poorly organized. The same label can hide very different realities.

Why Person-Level Explanations Come So Easily

Person-level explanations are attractive because they are simple. If someone is disorganized, weak, unprofessional, or unmotivated, the problem appears to be solved conceptually. The label feels like an answer. It also removes the need to ask what was happening around the learner. Simplicity can come at the cost of accuracy.

That problem becomes especially important in medical training because workplace-based judgments are shaped by what the assessor observes, the assessor's frame of reference, and the clinical context in which performance occurs (Govaerts et al., 2013). A supervisor may observe a learner on a difficult service, during a new workflow, or under conditions that are different from another rotation. The behavior still matters, but the context affects how it should be interpreted. A single setting can reveal a real weakness without telling you whether the weakness appears everywhere. Location requires more than identifying who received the feedback.

Environmental Problems Do Not Erase Learner Problems

Environmental problems do not erase learner responsibility. A humiliating feedback conversation can coexist with a genuine clinical reasoning problem. Inconsistent teaching can coexist with an ineffective study strategy. Poor supervision can make a problem harder to identify while the learner still needs to improve. Finding an environmental contribution does not settle the rest of the analysis.

The reverse is also true. A learner-level problem does not make the environment irrelevant. A student who is underprepared may still be receiving unclear expectations, and a resident who needs better communication skills may still be working in a team culture that discourages questions. Both parts matter because each may require a different response. The goal is to locate responsibility accurately enough that the right things can change.

If the learner needs to improve, that remains true even when the environment contributed. If the environment made the problem worse, that also deserves attention even when the learner has work to do.

That distinction helps prevent two common errors. Shame can pull the learner toward *everything is my fault*, while anger or fear can pull toward *the system did this to me*. Either conclusion may contain part of the truth. Neither feeling establishes causality. The evidence still has to do that work.

The Location Map

Take the setback and ask where each possible contributor sits. You are not trying to prove one side innocent or assign blame. You are trying to build a more accurate map of the problem. A useful map includes learner factors, environmental factors, and interaction factors. The point is to see which explanations deserve closer attention.

Learner

- Knowledge gap
- Weak study strategy
- Difficulty applying knowledge
- Poor follow-through
- Communication problem
- Clinical skill gap

Environment

- Unclear expectations
- Inconsistent supervision
- Excessive workload
- Poor feedback
- Limited opportunity for practice
- Structural barriers

Interaction

- New workflow plus weak prioritization
- Illness plus high workload
- Limited supervision plus an emerging skill gap
- Conflicting expectations plus difficulty asking for clarification

The categories are not meant to produce a perfect answer. They are meant to stop the analysis from collapsing too quickly into one explanation. A contributor can appear in more than one category depending on the situation. What matters is whether the location helps you understand what needs to be examined next. The map is a starting point, not a final diagnosis.

One question is worth adding at the end: **Which explanation am I most emotionally invested in being true?** A learner carrying shame may prefer the explanation that everything is their fault because it fits how they already feel. A learner who feels angry or threatened may prefer an explanation located entirely in the system. Emotional investment does not make an explanation wrong. It does make it worth checking against the evidence.

Research on learning environments gives us good reason to include workload and institutional conditions in the analysis of trainee functioning (Dyrbye et al., 2009; Dyrbye et al., 2021). Those findings do not tell us that the environment caused a particular learner's failed exam or difficult evaluation. They support a narrower conclusion: context belongs in the investigation. The person who receives the result is not automatically the entire cause of the result. **An outcome tells you where the problem became visible, not necessarily where it began.**

Chapter 5: Different Problems Need Different Solutions

After a setback, the instinct is often to respond with more effort. You study longer, add another resource, make a stricter schedule, or promise yourself that next time you will work harder. That response makes sense because effort has probably solved problems for you before. The difficulty is that effort does not tell you what went wrong. **Effort is not a diagnosis.**

Imagine two students who receive the same failing score. One did not know enough of the material, while the other knew it during untimed practice but could not retrieve it reliably on the exam. Their scores look the same on the page. The problems underneath them are different. Giving both students the same plan would miss that difference.

"I Failed" Is a Starting Point

A failed exam tells you that performance fell below the required standard. It does not tell you whether the problem involved knowledge, retrieval, study strategy, application, exhaustion, illness, or the conditions under which you were learning. A difficult clinical evaluation creates the same problem because similar ratings can arise from very different behaviors. The outcome tells you what needs investigation. It does not tell you what treatment to prescribe.

This is why simply increasing effort can fail. If your study method is poorly matched to the task, doubling the hours may give you twice as much exposure to the same ineffective method.

If your clinical reasoning is weak, reading more may help only if missing knowledge is actually the limiting problem. If expectations are unclear, extra preparation may still aim at the wrong target.

What Kind of Problem Is This?

It helps to sort possible problems into a few broad areas. These categories are a map for thinking, not a validated diagnostic system. They give you a way to ask better questions when the first explanation is too vague. Several categories may apply to the same setback. The purpose is to make the problem more specific.

Learning problems involve what you know and how you use it. You may have gaps in knowledge, trouble retrieving information, an ineffective learning strategy, or difficulty applying knowledge to unfamiliar cases. A student who recognizes material while reading may still struggle to recall it without prompts. Another may remember facts but have difficulty deciding which ones matter in a clinical problem. Those learners need different forms of practice.

Performance problems become visible while doing the work. They may involve clinical or procedural skills, communication, interpersonal functioning, professionalism, or performance under pressure. A resident may understand a patient's condition but give an unclear oral presentation. Another may know what to do but struggle to perform a procedure consistently. The visible problem needs to be described closely enough to show which skill is actually failing.

Capacity problems affect what you can currently execute. Exhaustion, illness, major life circumstances, and other demands can reduce the attention, time, or energy available for training. These factors may contribute to poor performance without fully explaining it. A real knowledge gap can coexist with severe exhaustion. Capacity belongs in the analysis because a plan that ignores it may be impossible to carry out.

Context problems arise from the conditions in which learning and performance occur. Feedback may be vague, supervision may be limited, expectations may shift between supervisors, or workload may leave little opportunity to practice the skill being assessed. These conditions can create problems or make existing weaknesses harder to recognize and correct. They also require a different response from a problem located mainly in the learner. Context should be examined with the same care as learner-level explanations.

Multiple difficulties can coexist. In one single-institution remediation program, most referred learners had more than one identified deficit, with medical knowledge, clinical reasoning, and professionalism among the most common concerns (Guerrasio et al., 2014). That makes a single explanation less likely to fit every case. It also explains why broad advice such as *study harder* or *be more confident* is often inadequate. Real setbacks are frequently more complicated than the first label suggests.

Look for More Than One Contributor

Searching for one cause can become frustrating when several things went wrong together. A student may have weak foundations, rely on passive review, sleep poorly, and lose additional study time to a family crisis. A resident may need stronger clinical reasoning while also receiving inconsistent supervision on a high-volume service. Choosing one explanation too early can hide the others. The better question is which contributors matter enough to address.

This also keeps investigation from turning into endless self-analysis. You do not need a perfect explanation for every decision that led to the setback. You need an explanation good enough to guide the next useful test. If changing one suspected contributor improves performance, that gives you new evidence. If nothing changes, you revise the explanation.

The sequence is practical: develop a good-enough explanation, test it, and update it when necessary. This approach leaves room for complexity without requiring complete certainty. You can act while some questions remain open. The next action should help you learn more about the problem. Investigation earns its value by changing what you do.

A Correct Explanation Can Still Be Too Shallow

Sometimes the first explanation is accurate but incomplete. Saying *I failed because I did not know the material* may describe what happened on the exam. It still leaves open why the knowledge gap developed. Perhaps the foundations were weak, the study method was ineffective, illness interrupted preparation, or avoidance after an earlier poor result reduced the time spent on difficult material. **A correct diagnosis can still be too shallow.**

The same problem appears in clinical training. A resident may genuinely have trouble prioritizing a differential diagnosis. The next question is whether the problem comes from missing knowledge, difficulty organizing information, insufficient practice, uncertainty under observation, or another contributor. Knowing that reasoning is weak identifies the area that needs work. Understanding why it is weak helps determine what kind of work is likely to help.

You do not always need to keep digging further upstream. If a clear skill gap has an obvious intervention and improvement follows, further causal analysis may add little. More investigation becomes useful when the first intervention fails or when the same difficulty keeps returning. The depth of the explanation should match the decision you need to make. The purpose is useful understanding, not complete reconstruction of the past.

Build a Differential, Not a Defense

After a painful result, explanations can become emotionally loaded. *I did not work hard enough* may feel appropriately self-critical, while *the exam was unfair* may feel protective. Either explanation could contain useful information. Neither deserves to win simply because it feels more responsible or more comforting. Treat each explanation as a hypothesis that needs evidence.

This is similar to the logic used in clinical reasoning. A physician does not choose a diagnosis because it is the most emotionally satisfying possibility. Plausible explanations are considered, evidence is gathered, and the list changes as new information arrives. Remediation scholarship uses a related sequence by emphasizing detection of a difficulty, collection of objective information, development of an educational diagnosis, and a targeted plan (Boileau et al., 2017). Here, the learner can use the same discipline on their own setback.

The Setback Differential

Choose one visible problem and work through the following prompts.

Visible problem

What happened?

Possible explanations

What are two or three plausible reasons this could have happened?

Supporting evidence

What makes each explanation plausible?

Contradictory evidence

What facts do not fit each explanation?

Missing information

What do you still need to know?

Next useful test

What could you do or find out that would help distinguish among the explanations?

For example, suppose the visible problem is failing a pharmacology exam. One explanation is inadequate knowledge, supported by weak scores across several content areas. Another is poor retrieval, supported by being able to recognize answers while reviewing but struggling to recall information without prompts. A third is disrupted preparation during illness, supported by a substantial loss of study time in the weeks before the exam. The next useful test might include reviewing the score breakdown and completing a short set of closed-book questions before choosing a new study plan.

The exercise is meant to narrow the next decision. You do not need to prove exactly how much each factor contributed. You need enough evidence to choose an intervention that fits the most important problem. If the intervention works, you have learned something about the explanation. If it does not, the explanation deserves another look.

A setback can make harder work feel like the safest response. Hard work matters, but it becomes much more useful when you know what the work is supposed to change. **The purpose is not perfect causal certainty. The purpose is choosing a better next action.**

Chapter 6: Evidence Before Explanation

After a setback, explanations come quickly. One attending thought your reasoning was weak, one exam score was below passing, or one meeting ended with concerns about your progress. The temptation is to decide what those events mean before asking how strong the evidence actually is. Some information deserves substantial weight, while other information should remain provisional. The task is to judge the evidence before building too much around it.

That matters because difficult feedback can pull in opposite directions. You may want to dismiss it because it hurts, or you may give it more authority because it hurts. Neither response tells you whether the information is accurate. How much feedback hurts and how much evidence it carries have to be judged separately. A painful evaluation can be important without being automatically right.

Not All Evidence Carries the Same Weight

Evidence differs in how specific, direct, consistent, and relevant it is. One vague sentence in an evaluation is different from three supervisors independently describing the same behavior. A comment from someone who worked with you twice is different from repeated observations across several weeks. A general impression is different from a description of what you actually did. These differences should change how much confidence you place in the conclusion.

Consider the comment *needs more confidence*. It may reflect something real, but the phrase tells you very little about the underlying behavior. Did the learner hesitate before committing to a plan, speak quietly, ask for reassurance, or change answers when challenged? Each of those behaviors could have a different explanation. The more clearly the behavior is described, the more useful the evidence becomes.

Direct observation also matters. A supervisor who watched you present several patients has more information about your presentations than someone who heard about them secondhand. A preceptor who observed one brief interaction may still identify something important, but the scope of the claim should match the opportunity to observe. Limited observation does not make feedback worthless. It places limits on what the feedback can establish.

Two Ways to Misread Difficult Evidence

Painful information is easy to discount. You may decide that the evaluator was unfair, the exam was poorly written, or the feedback was too vague to matter. Sometimes those concerns are justified. Sometimes they become a way of avoiding information that needs attention. Discomfort alone does not make the evidence weak.

The opposite error is just as common. A harsh comment may feel more credible because it matches your worst fear about yourself. You may assume that if the feedback was painful enough to upset you, it must contain some deeper truth. That conclusion gives emotion more authority than observation. Pain does not make evidence stronger either.

A painful evaluation may contain important information, or it may turn out to be poorly supported. How much it hurts does not help you decide between those possibilities.

The useful question is what supports it. Who observed the behavior, what did they see, how often did it occur, and does the same pattern appear elsewhere? Those questions do more work than deciding whether the feedback felt fair. They move the analysis back toward evidence.

Questions That Increase or Decrease Confidence

A few questions can help establish how much weight a concern deserves. Was the feedback based on direct observation, and were specific behaviors described? Did the evaluator have enough opportunity to see the skill being judged? Were the expectations clear before the assessment? Stronger answers to those questions usually give the information more weight.

Convergence matters too. If several supervisors who worked with you independently describe the same difficulty, the concern deserves more attention. If one supervisor reports a problem while several others describe strong performance in the same area, that contradiction also matters. Neither pattern settles the question automatically. It tells you what should be examined next.

Context can change interpretation without erasing the result. Poor performance during a period of illness may still be poor performance, while illness may affect what the result tells you about usual functioning. A weak evaluation on one unusually chaotic service may identify a real vulnerability that becomes visible only under certain conditions. That can still be useful information. The question is how broadly the evidence should be generalized.

Standards also matter. Feedback is easier to judge when the learner knows what level of performance was expected. A comment that someone is "not efficient enough" carries less information when no one has defined what adequate efficiency looks like. A specific standard allows the learner to compare behavior with an expectation instead of guessing what the evaluator meant. Clear standards make evidence easier to interpret.

What Do the Common Cases Actually Tell You?

One poor evaluation is worth examining, but it does not automatically establish a pattern. You need to know how much the evaluator observed, what behaviors were described, and whether similar concerns appear elsewhere. One isolated concern may remain important, especially if the behavior was serious. Its scope should still remain narrow until more evidence is available. One data point becomes stronger when other independent evidence points in the same direction.

One failed exam also deserves attention without answering every question about future performance. The score may reveal important weaknesses, but its meaning depends partly on what the score breakdown shows and whether similar problems have appeared before. A pattern across several assessments carries more weight than one unexpected result. Context such as illness or severe disruption may also affect interpretation. The next step is to determine what the exam actually tells you and what remains unknown.

Repeated feedback deserves a different response. If three supervisors independently describe difficulty prioritizing the differential, the concern is harder to dismiss as one person's impression. You still need to understand exactly what each person observed and whether the same behavior appeared under similar conditions. Repetition strengthens the case that there is something worth addressing. It also helps narrow what needs work.

Vague feedback creates a different problem because there may not be enough information to act. *Needs more confidence* or *should be more professional* can leave the learner guessing about what behavior needs to change. The appropriate next step may be clarification rather than self-correction based on assumptions.

Ask for examples, situations, and the standard that was expected. Evidence that cannot yet guide action may simply need to become more specific.

Suspected bias also requires careful investigation, and the possibility should not be treated as merely a defensive explanation. Medical-education research has documented bias and disparities in clinical assessment related to characteristics including race, ethnicity, and gender, although evidence of disparities at the group level does not establish the cause of any single evaluation (Hauer et al., 2023; Ismaeel et al., 2024). For an individual evaluation, look at the behavior described, the assessor's opportunity to observe it, patterns across evaluators and settings, and whether similar differences in language or scoring recur. The aim is not to assume either discrimination or deficiency. It is to investigate both possibilities seriously enough that neither is dismissed in advance.

Enough Evidence to Act

You rarely need complete certainty before taking a useful next step. If several sources point to the same communication problem, you may have enough information to seek direct observation and targeted practice. If the evidence is mixed, you may need another observer before committing to a broad explanation. If the feedback is too vague, clarification itself may be the next action. Action can begin before every question is settled.

This matters because searching for perfect certainty can become another form of delay. You may never know exactly how much each factor contributed to a failed exam or difficult rotation. The practical question is whether the evidence is strong enough to guide what happens next. A good next step should also generate more information. Useful action and better evidence can develop together.

Learners do not simply receive feedback and accept it without interpretation. Research has shown that learners make judgments about the credibility and meaning of performance information, and that feedback depends on interactions between the learner and the surrounding environment rather than simple transmission alone (Watling et al., 2012; Watling, 2014). Extending that reasoning to how learners interpret setbacks more broadly is a synthesis used in this book. The same discipline applies: ask what the evidence supports before deciding how much the event should mean. You need enough evidence to choose the next reasonable action. You do not need one evaluation, one score, or one explanation to answer every larger question about your future.

The Evidence Check

Take one explanation you currently believe and ask five questions.

- What evidence supports it?
- How direct and specific is that evidence?
- Do independent sources point in the same direction?
- What evidence does not fit?
- What new information would change my mind?

The goal is not to win an argument with yourself. It is to find out how confident you should be in the explanation you are using. Some explanations will become stronger after this review, while others will become more tentative. Both outcomes are useful. The next step should follow the evidence, not the intensity of the fear.

You do not need perfect causal certainty before acting. You need enough evidence to choose a reasonable next step and enough openness to revise the explanation when new information appears. That is the point of Part II: locate the problem, consider plausible explanations, and test them against what you actually know. Better evidence makes the next action less arbitrary. **The**

purpose is not certainty. The purpose is a better-informed response.

Part III: Getting Functioning Back

Understanding the problem does not automatically make you able to act on it. You may know what needs to change and still hesitate, avoid the work, overthink each step, or wait to feel more confident before beginning. Exhaustion or the conditions around you may also make a reasonable plan hard to carry out. The next problem is practical: becoming able to respond.

That usually happens before confidence is fully restored. You may return to the question bank while still anxious, ask for feedback while still embarrassed, or change a study plan before you know whether it will work. The next chapters focus on the barriers that interfere with that movement, including avoidance, self-condemnation, ineffective persistence, limited capacity, and trying to recover alone. Each problem calls for a different response. The organizing principle is simple: **function before confidence.**

The work now is to re-enter what you have been avoiding, take responsibility for what is yours, redesign what is not working, and make sure the plan can fit the life and training environment you actually have. Other people may need to be part of that process, whether they provide information, coaching, advocacy, or simple steadiness. Progress will come from acting, then looking again at what the evidence shows. You do not need to rebuild everything at once. You need the next workable step.

Chapter 7: Avoidance Makes Sense and Still Has a Cost

After a setback, ordinary tasks can start to feel different. The question bank is no longer just a place to practice, the evaluation portal is no longer just a website, and the simulation lab is no longer just a place to learn. Each one may now feel like a test of whether the fear is true. Opening the task can feel like opening the possibility of another failure. That change in meaning can make avoidance surprisingly easy to understand.

You may delay reading the score report, postpone contacting a supervisor, or spend hours on work that feels safer than the problem in front of you. From the outside, this can look like procrastination or poor follow-through. Sometimes that is exactly what it is. Other times, the task has become tied to embarrassment, uncertainty, or fear about what it might reveal. **Sometimes you are avoiding the work because of what you fear the work will tell you.**

Why Avoidance Works at First

Avoidance persists because it usually works in the short term. When you close the evaluation portal, postpone the meeting, or decide not to look at the weak content area tonight, discomfort often drops. Research on procrastination has described this short-term mood repair as one reason people delay difficult tasks despite later costs (Sirois & Pychyl, 2013). Applying that idea specifically to avoidance after a training setback is used here.

The immediate relief is real even when the longer-term result is worse.

That short-term relief can make avoidance feel like recovery. For an hour, you are no longer looking at the score, thinking about the supervisor, or confronting the material that went badly. The problem is still waiting when the relief passes. Sometimes it has also grown because a deadline is closer, useful information is still missing, or preparation time has been lost. What helped for ten minutes can make tomorrow harder.

One plausible cycle is that a setback makes the task more threatening, and avoiding the task then reduces practice or delays information. That can increase uncertainty and, in some situations, leave the learner less prepared for the next attempt. Avoidance can therefore begin contributing to some of the evidence the learner was afraid of finding. This is one possible pathway after a setback, not an explanation for every repeated difficulty.

That cycle does not mean the original concern was imaginary. You may have a real knowledge gap, a serious performance problem, or consequences that need attention. Avoidance does not create every difficulty that follows a setback. It can still make a real problem harder to assess and correct. That short-term relief is worth understanding, but it should not determine the plan.

The Task Changed

A useful question is what the task means now that did not mean before. Before the failed exam, opening the question bank may have meant *I am going to practice cardiology*. Afterward, it may mean *I am about to find out whether I am still failing*. The question bank itself has not changed. What opening it now seems to mean has.

The same thing can happen with feedback. Before a difficult rotation, asking a supervisor for comments may have felt routine. After one concerning evaluation, the same conversation may feel like an opportunity for someone to confirm your worst fear. You may begin avoiding feedback at exactly the point when better feedback would be most useful. The task becomes threatening because of the meaning attached to the answer.

This distinction does not excuse indefinite delay. If an email is due, it still needs to be sent, and a remediation requirement still has to be completed. It does explain why a task that used to be easy to begin may now take much more effort. Calling that difficulty laziness may add shame without improving the response. Understanding what changed gives you a better place to intervene.

Do Not Wait Until the Task Feels Safe

A common re-entry rule is *I will start when I feel ready*. After a threatening setback, that condition may keep moving because readiness is being measured by the absence of fear. You wait for the question bank to stop making you anxious, the meeting to stop feeling threatening, or the clinical setting to feel normal again. Those feelings may improve only after you have had new experiences with the task. Waiting can therefore make the task remain unfamiliar and threatening.

Re-entry usually works better when it is smaller than the full task. You do not need to complete two hours of practice to begin approaching the question bank again. You might open the score report, identify one weak domain, and stop there. You might draft the email before deciding when to send it. A useful first encounter should be small enough to complete while still moving you toward the problem.

You do not have to make the task comfortable before approaching it. Make the first encounter small enough to complete and useful enough to teach you something about what happens next. A small step can show you that the task is possible while also revealing what remains difficult. That evidence is more useful than waiting to feel completely confident. **Function can begin before confidence returns.**

The Re-Entry Ladder

Start by naming the task you are avoiding. Be concrete enough that you can picture the action, such as opening the written evaluation, completing ten questions from the failed content area, or scheduling the meeting with the course director. Then ask what the task has come to represent. The answer may be another failure, humiliation, bad news, or evidence that you still do not understand the material. Knowing what you fear helps explain why the task feels larger than it looks.

Next, identify the smallest useful encounter with the task. Reading the first paragraph of an evaluation may be enough for one step, while answering five questions without checking the score until the end may be enough for another. Decide what would make that encounter possible, such as choosing a quiet time, asking someone to sit nearby, or clarifying what information you are trying to obtain. Then look for evidence that you are ready for the next step. The ladder should increase contact with the task without turning each step into another test of worth.

A re-entry ladder might look like this:

- Open the score report and read it once.
- Identify the two weakest domains.
- Complete five questions from one weak domain.
- Review the errors without changing the study plan yet.
- Complete another short set two days later.
- Review the pattern and decide what needs to change.

The steps should remain useful even if they feel uncomfortable. If the first step is so small that it does not bring you into contact with the problem, it may simply become another form of delay. If the first step is so large that you repeatedly cannot begin it, make the step smaller. Each step needs to be small enough that you can do it and large enough that it actually brings you back into contact with the problem.

Sometimes the Conditions Need to Change First

Re-entry is not the right answer to every form of avoidance. A learner who is acutely ill, working under unsafe supervision, experiencing ongoing mistreatment, or waiting for an essential accommodation may need a change in conditions before more exposure to the task is useful. The same is true when workload is structurally unmanageable. Pushing harder in those circumstances can individualize a problem that requires another kind of response. Sometimes the barrier is the environment, not reluctance to face the work.

This boundary matters because perseverance is easy to overvalue in training. A student may assume that continuing despite illness proves commitment, or a resident may believe tolerating unsafe conditions is part of becoming tougher. Those assumptions can make any pause look like avoidance. The useful question is what the pause is doing. A pause that increases your ability to respond is different from one that allows the problem to grow.

Strategic Delay, Stabilization, and Avoidance

Not every delay is avoidance. Sometimes waiting produces a better decision because important information will soon be available. If the written policy is released tomorrow, delaying an appeal decision until you can read it may be sensible. That is strategic delay because the wait improves the quality of the next action. The delay has a reason and an endpoint.

Stabilization is different again. You may need a bounded period to sleep, attend to an urgent health problem, arrange childcare, or regain enough capacity to have a useful conversation. The pause is serving the next action rather than replacing it. Its purpose is to improve your ability to respond. A stabilization period should make the next step more possible.

Avoidance usually has a different effect. The delay reduces discomfort now while leaving the important task unchanged or making it harder later. The email remains unsent, the deadline gets closer, or the weak material remains untouched. There may be no clear plan for when or how the task will be approached. The relief is immediate, but the problem grows.

A useful question can separate these situations:

Is this pause increasing my capacity to respond, or allowing the problem to grow?

The answer may not be obvious at first. A night away from studying may be stabilization for one learner and avoidance for another. The difference lies in what the pause is for, whether it has boundaries, and what happens next. Looking at the function of the delay is more useful than judging yourself for taking it.

Re-Entry Before Readiness

You do not need to feel certain before you begin again. The first email can be sent while you are still embarrassed, and the first practice set can happen while you are still afraid of the score. Those feelings may remain present for a while. Waiting for them to disappear can hand them control over the timing of your recovery. A small useful action can happen before the emotional part catches up.

The same principle applies when the first attempt goes badly. You may open the question bank and still miss several items, or attend the meeting and leave with more work than you hoped for. That does not make the re-entry a failure. The purpose of re-entry is to make contact with the problem and learn from what happens.

Avoidance makes sense because it can reduce discomfort quickly. Its cost is that the information, practice, or conversation you need remains on the other side of the task. Recovery rarely begins when the work finally feels harmless. It begins when you can approach something useful despite the discomfort that remains. **Function before confidence.**

Chapter 8: Accountability Without Self-Condemnation

Sometimes the investigation leads somewhere uncomfortable. You may discover that you did not prepare adequately, ignored feedback, handled a responsibility poorly, or made a mistake that had consequences. At that point, explanations about workload, supervision, or circumstances may matter without changing the central fact that something was yours to correct. This is often where responsibility gets confused with punishment. If you believe being hard on yourself is what keeps you accountable, describing the problem without attacking yourself can feel suspiciously lenient.

Accountability asks what happened, what part was yours, and what needs to change. Self-condemnation turns the same information into a judgment about the kind of person you are. The first can lead to action because it keeps the problem specific. The second often makes the problem larger while giving you less direction. You do not need to humiliate yourself to take a mistake seriously.

The False Choice

Medical training can make self-criticism feel useful. If you believe harshness keeps you disciplined, then easing up on yourself may feel dangerously close to making excuses. You may worry that saying *I made a mistake* is too gentle unless it becomes *I am careless*. The fear underneath is understandable: if I stop attacking myself, maybe I will stop improving. That assumption deserves a closer look.

The choice is not between self-condemnation and pretending nothing happened. You can acknowledge that your preparation was inadequate without deciding that you are lazy. You can accept that your communication caused a problem without deciding that you are an inconsiderate person. You can recognize that you missed an important clinical finding without reassuring yourself that it did not matter. Responsibility becomes clearer when it stays attached to what actually happened.

Accountability Names the Problem

Specific language makes accountability more demanding, not less. *I underestimated how much practice I needed and relied too heavily on passive review* identifies choices that can be changed. *I am lazy* offers a harsher description with very little instructional value. One statement points toward a new plan, while the other points back toward the self. **Accountability becomes more actionable as it becomes more specific.**

The same distinction applies to clinical work. *I did not review the medication changes before handoff, and I left out an important update* tells you what failed. You can decide how the handoff process needs to change and how to reduce the chance of repeating the omission. *I am irresponsible* may feel like a fuller admission because it hurts more. Pain is not what makes an explanation accurate.

This does not mean every mistake can be reduced to one isolated behavior. Repeated actions may eventually establish a pattern that deserves broader concern. Someone who repeatedly ignores deadlines, dismisses feedback, or behaves disrespectfully may need to examine more than one incident. Even then, describing the pattern precisely remains more useful than reaching immediately for a character label. A pattern can be serious without becoming an explanation of the entire person.

When "I Did" Becomes "I Am"

Shame can change the focus of a setback. Earlier, we separated disappointment about an event from the global conclusion that the problem is the self. That distinction becomes especially important when there really is something to take responsibility for. The presence of responsibility can make self-condemnation feel deserved. It does not make self-condemnation more useful.

Suppose you failed because you did far less active practice than you knew the course required. You may need to acknowledge that you made a poor decision about preparation and that the consequences are yours to deal with. Calling yourself lazy adds another claim that now requires evidence about your behavior across time and settings. It also gives you no clear instruction for what to do differently tomorrow. Accountability works best when the description stays close to the behavior.

Research on shame distinguishes global negative evaluation of the self from responses focused more closely on actions, and medical-education research has described how shame can threaten learners' sense of worth and belonging (Bynum et al., 2019; Bynum et al., 2021b; Tangney & Dearing, 2002). These findings do not mean that every strong negative reaction after a mistake is shame. They do support paying attention to the point where criticism shifts from *what I did* to *what I am*. That shift can make correction harder to see. The behavior still needs attention even when the global judgment does not help.

Self-Compassion Is Not Self-Reassurance

Self-compassion is sometimes mistaken for telling yourself that everything is fine. That would be reassurance, and reassurance may be inaccurate when a serious problem has occurred. A more useful response sounds different: *This is painful, and I may have made a significant mistake. I can examine what happened without using humiliation as my method of improvement.* The difficulty remains in the picture.

Research on self-compassion does not support the simple claim that treating yourself less harshly removes motivation to improve. Work by Neff (2003) describes self-compassion as a way of responding to personal difficulty, while experimental work by Breines and Chen (2012) found that self-compassion can coexist with motivation for self-improvement. Those findings do not establish that self-compassion improves outcomes in medical training. They support the narrower point that self-compassion and corrective motivation are not inherently incompatible. You do not have to choose between taking yourself seriously and treating yourself decently.

Self-compassion also does not decide whether you were responsible. Evidence does that work. If you ignored repeated feedback, self-compassion does not turn the feedback into someone else's problem. If the environment contributed, self-criticism does not make the environment disappear. Self-compassion changes how responsibility is carried after the evidence has been examined.

What Is Actually Yours?

Responsibility is often easier to manage when it is divided into parts. A setback may contain behavior that clearly belongs to you, circumstances that were outside your control, and areas where responsibility was shared. Putting everything in one category usually distorts the problem. Taking too much responsibility can produce shame, while taking too little can block change. Accurate responsibility gives each part somewhere to go.

Imagine a student who failed after studying inconsistently during a period of serious family disruption. The student may genuinely have avoided difficult material and used an ineffective study method. The family situation may also have reduced available time and concentration in ways that were not chosen. A useful account includes both pieces without using one to cancel the other. The question is what the student can learn from each part.

The same reasoning applies when the environment was clearly problematic. A resident may have received humiliating feedback from a supervisor and still have interrupted team members repeatedly during rounds. The supervisor's behavior may require institutional attention, while the resident's communication may also need work. One problem does not erase the other. Accuracy means refusing to use either problem as a reason to ignore the second one.

The Accountability Audit

Take one setback and answer the following questions as concretely as possible.

What happened?

Describe the event without adding a character judgment.

What part is mine?

Identify choices, behaviors, preparation, or follow-through that you reasonably own.

What is not mine alone?

Identify circumstances, supervision, workload, unclear expectations, or other contributors that also belong in the explanation.

What will I do differently?

Name one or two changes that directly address your part of the problem.

What am I calling myself?

Write down the labels you have attached to yourself, then ask whether each label adds information that the behavioral description does not.

The audit is not designed to divide responsibility perfectly. In many situations, you will not know exactly how much each contributor mattered. The purpose is to identify enough responsibility to guide action without claiming responsibility for everything that happened. It also makes excuses easier to see because genuine ownership has to be named explicitly. **Explanation is not exemption.**

Accountability May Include Consequences

Taking responsibility does not guarantee that the consequence disappears. You may have to repeat an assessment, complete supervised practice, enter remediation, or accept closer monitoring for a period of time. Progression may be delayed because competence has not yet been demonstrated. If your actions harmed someone, accountability may also require acknowledging that harm or apologizing. These consequences can be appropriate even when you understand why the problem happened.

Consequences and shame answer different questions. A repeated assessment addresses whether you can meet the required standard. Supervised practice addresses whether a skill needs further development before independent performance. An apology addresses harm that occurred in a relationship. Calling yourself a failure does none of those jobs. **Consequences answer what needs to happen next. Shame tries to answer what kind of person you are.**

Accepting a consequence can be especially difficult when you already understand what went wrong. You may think that insight should be enough to prove the problem has been fixed. In medical training, understanding a problem and demonstrating corrected performance are different things. A program may reasonably require new evidence before changing its assessment. Accountability includes producing that evidence when it is required.

What Changes Now?

Once your part of the problem is clear enough, further self-criticism adds little. The useful question becomes what will change because you understand the problem differently. Maybe you will begin practice earlier, ask for direct observation, create a better handoff routine, or respond to feedback before the same concern appears again. The action should be tied closely to the problem you identified. Improvement becomes easier to evaluate when the change is concrete.

This is also where endless confession can become another form of avoidance. Repeatedly telling yourself how badly you handled something may feel like taking responsibility while allowing you to postpone the harder work of changing the behavior. Remorse can matter, especially when harm occurred. It still has to lead somewhere. Accountability becomes visible in what happens next.

The question after a setback is not how to avoid responsibility. It is how to identify what is yours and respond to it usefully. Some of what happened may be yours, and some of it may carry consequences that you would rather not face. You can accept those facts without turning them into a complete judgment about yourself. **Accountability names what needs to change and leaves the rest of the person available to do the changing.**

Chapter 9: Redesign, Not Rededication

After a setback, many trainees respond by promising to work harder. You add hours, resources, flashcards, question blocks, and stricter rules for yourself. The new plan may look different because it is more demanding. If the underlying problem has not changed, the plan may still be doing the same thing. **A more punishing version of the same plan is still the same plan.**

Effort matters, and there are times when more practice is exactly what is needed. The problem is that effort is nonspecific, so it cannot tell you which part of the system needs to change. Someone with a knowledge gap needs a different response from someone who knows the material but cannot apply it to cases. Someone struggling with an unclear clinical standard needs something different again. **Persistence without diagnosis can become repetition.**

Start With the Problem You Actually Found

A useful redesign begins with the explanation that survived the investigation. If the problem is missing knowledge, the plan should build the missing knowledge. If retrieval is weak, the learner needs repeated practice recalling information without prompts. If the problem appears during clinical application, more case-based reasoning and coached practice may be more useful than another pass through the textbook. The intervention should match the problem closely enough that you would expect it to help.

Clinical and performance problems require the same discipline. A procedural skill gap calls for observation, practice, and feedback on the skill itself. Unclear expectations call for clarification, while poor feedback may require more direct observation from someone able to describe the behavior precisely. Excessive demand may require changes in workload or in the conditions under which the recovery plan is expected to run. Remediation guidance similarly favors targeted plans based on the identified difficulty rather than generic repetition (Audétat et al., 2013; Kalet et al., 2016).

The plan should also help test the explanation that produced it. If you believe weak retrieval contributed to the failed exam, a period of closed-book recall practice should produce evidence about whether retrieval improves. If the suspected problem is organization during oral presentations, a more structured presentation approach should be observable to you and your supervisors. When the expected change does not appear, the explanation may need revision. **The intervention should reveal whether the diagnosis was right.**

Change One Important Thing

A setback can create an urge to rebuild everything at once. You buy new resources, make a new schedule, find a tutor, change your study method, alter your sleep routine, and reorganize the rest of your life. The plan feels serious because nearly every part of it is new. A few weeks later, it may be impossible to tell which changes helped or why the plan became difficult to maintain. Total reinvention can create activity without producing much useful evidence.

A smaller experiment is often easier to learn from. Begin with one explanation about what is limiting performance, then change something directly related to it. Decide in advance what evidence would suggest the change is helping, and review that evidence after a defined period. Keep the change if it appears useful, and revise the explanation if it does not. **Treat redesign as hypothesis testing instead of self-reinvention.**

Suppose you failed an exam and concluded that passive review left you recognizing material without being able to retrieve it. For the next two weeks, you replace part of the rereading with closed-book questions and active recall in the two weakest domains. You track whether you can retrieve the material later and whether performance improves on new questions. At the review point, you decide whether retrieval is improving enough to continue the approach. The experiment gives you more information than simply adding another three hours to each study day.

Decide What Improvement Would Look Like

A redesign is hard to evaluate if improvement is described only as a feeling. *I want to feel more confident* may matter personally, but confidence can rise or fall for reasons that have little to do with competence. A clearer indicator is something you or another person can observe. You might answer a higher proportion of new questions correctly, complete notes within the expected time, or consistently include contingency plans in handoffs. Observable changes give the redesign something concrete to produce.

Clinical goals become more useful when they describe behavior. *Be better at presentations* is vague, while *state the problem representation before giving the differential and prioritize the top three diagnoses* can be observed. *Be more confident with procedures* is difficult to measure, while *complete each step of the procedure with decreasing prompting across three supervised attempts* gives you something to review. The indicator does not need to capture everything that matters. It needs to show whether the targeted problem is changing.

This also protects against judging the plan by mood alone. You may be improving while still feeling anxious, or feel more comfortable without showing much change in performance. Neither feeling should be ignored, but neither is enough by itself to evaluate the redesign. The question is what evidence was supposed to change and whether it did. **If you cannot observe the change, you cannot reliably evaluate the redesign.**

Act First, Then Review

Once the experiment begins, give yourself enough room to perform it. Every practice question does not need to become a judgment about whether the entire recovery plan is working. One difficult study session does not prove the intervention has failed, and one excellent session does not prove the problem is solved. Practice will contain ordinary variation. You need enough data to see a pattern.

Choose a review point before you begin. At that point, ask what changed, what stayed the same, and what new evidence appeared. If the expected improvement occurred, continue or build on the intervention. If the outcome stayed flat, decide whether the change was too small, poorly executed, or aimed at the wrong problem. The review is where interpretation belongs.

This protects against the self-surveillance that can follow a setback. A missed question can remain a missed question instead of becoming evidence that you are still failing. An anxious presentation can remain one uncomfortable presentation instead of deciding whether you are ready to continue. The experiment needs repeated observations more than repeated conclusions. **Do the planned work, then review what the pattern shows.**

When the New Plan Does Not Work

A failed redesign is still information. If you change the study strategy and performance does not improve, the original explanation may have been incomplete. If repeated coached practice does not change a clinical behavior, another contributor may be limiting progress. The answer may be a different intervention, more observation, or a deeper look at what is driving the difficulty. An unsuccessful plan can move the investigation forward if you use it as evidence.

Sometimes several reasonable interventions fail. Repeated difficulty despite targeted practice, adequate support, and clear expectations may eventually provide meaningful information about a learner's limitations. That possibility should not be hidden simply because it is uncomfortable. Some goals, timelines, specialties, or training paths may eventually need to change. Those decisions deserve more evidence than the intensity of the original setback.

This is another reason to avoid changing everything at once. When ten variables change together, a poor result tells you very little about which part of the plan failed. A focused redesign creates cleaner information even when it does not produce the outcome you wanted. Each round should leave you knowing something you did not know before. Recovery becomes a series of informed adjustments rather than repeated acts of recommitment.

The Redesign Canvas

Use one page to connect the explanation with the next action.

Diagnosis

What problem are you currently trying to change?

Intervention

What specific change addresses that problem?

Observable indicator

What would you expect to see if the intervention is helping?

Review point

When will you stop and examine the evidence?

Decision rule

What will make you continue, modify, or stop the intervention?

A redesign should be small enough to run and specific enough to evaluate. If the plan requires an entirely new life before it can succeed, the plan may be too large. If you cannot say what evidence would show that it is working, the intervention may still be too vague. Make one meaningful change, then learn from what follows. A good plan produces information as well as effort.

Working harder can feel like the most responsible response to a setback. Sometimes the correct redesign will indeed require more practice, more preparation, or more deliberate effort. The difference is that the additional work now has a target and a way to judge whether it is helping. When the evidence changes, the plan can change with it. **Recovery requires more than rededication when the original approach was part of the problem.**

Chapter 10: Recovery Has Infrastructure

A good plan can fail because the system expected to carry it cannot support it. Imagine a resident with a careful remediation plan built around regular practice, reflection, and feedback while working rotating nights, carrying an intense service, and commuting an hour each way. The plan may be reasonable on paper and impossible in practice. When it breaks down, the resident may conclude that discipline is the problem. Sometimes the plan simply asks more than the learner's current life can support.

That distinction matters because recovery is often discussed as though it depends mainly on motivation. Motivation can matter, but it cannot create time, sleep, supervision, transportation, childcare, or a manageable workload. A learner can be fully committed and still have too little capacity to execute a demanding plan reliably. The same learner may perform very differently when those conditions change. A recovery plan has to fit the system around it.

Capacity Is Not Character

Capacity describes what you can currently carry. It can be affected by workload, illness, sleep, caregiving, stress, and the number of competing demands that require attention. Sustained demands can impose cumulative physiological costs over time, which is one reason prolonged strain belongs in the background of any discussion about functioning (McEwen, 1998). That does not tell us why a particular learner struggled. It does remind us that human performance has limits.

Those limits are easy to moralize in training. If you cannot sustain twelve-hour study days after a difficult rotation, you may decide that you are weak. If you cannot complete a complicated recovery plan while working nights, you may decide that you lack discipline. Those conclusions convert a capacity problem into a character judgment. A more useful question is what the current system can realistically support.

Capacity can also change over time. A learner who is ill, grieving, pregnant, caregiving, or severely exhausted may have less available capacity for a period without having permanently lost professional potential. That current limit can still matter because standards do not disappear simply because circumstances are difficult. The question is whether the limit is temporary, modifiable, accommodated, or evidence of a more persistent mismatch. **Capacity is real even when it is temporary.**

What Recovery Depends On

Recovery rarely runs on effort alone. It depends on a set of practical conditions that make action possible. Some are personal, some are educational, and some are institutional. When one part fails, the entire plan may become harder to carry out. Looking at the infrastructure can reveal why an otherwise sensible plan keeps breaking down.

Physiological conditions matter because sleep, illness, nutrition, and treatment affect what a learner can sustain. Cognitive conditions matter because protected time, interruptions, and competing demands determine whether focused work can actually happen. Logistical conditions such as childcare, housing, finances, transportation, and commute time can shape how much room is left for recovery. Educational conditions include direct observation, coaching, clear expectations, and accommodations when appropriate. Relational and institutional conditions matter because supervision, policy clarity, psychological safety, and remediation structures can either support or obstruct the work.

No learner needs every condition to be ideal before improvement is possible. Medical training rarely offers ideal conditions, and some adaptation is always required. The point is to identify which constraints are significant enough to affect whether the plan can work. A recovery strategy that ignores those constraints may look ambitious while remaining fragile. **The plan has to fit the life that actually exists.**

When "Self-Care" Misses the Problem

Advice about self-care can become unhelpful when the main problem is structural. Telling a resident to sleep more while scheduling repeated overnight shifts does not address the schedule. Telling a student to reduce stress while leaving unclear expectations and conflicting deadlines unchanged may place responsibility in the wrong place. Individual habits still matter, but they cannot correct every environmental problem. Some conditions require changes outside the learner.

The opposite error is also possible. A difficult environment can become an explanation for behavior that is still within the learner's control. A heavy workload does not automatically explain repeated failure to respond to clear messages, and inconsistent teaching does not make an ineffective study strategy irrelevant. The environment should not be used to avoid changes that genuinely belong to the learner. Accurate recovery requires locating which part of the problem each intervention is supposed to address.

These distinctions prevent "capacity" from becoming another vague label. A plan may fail because the learner is temporarily depleted, because an accommodation is missing, because the workload is unrealistic, or because the learner has a genuine competence gap. Those are different problems and should not be collapsed into one category. The task is to identify which limit is operating and what kind of response fits it. **Do not prescribe individual adaptation for a problem that primarily requires environmental change.**

Is the Plan Realistic?

A recovery plan should be tested against the learner's actual schedule. A plan that requires three uninterrupted study hours every evening may fail if the learner is on call, commuting, or caring for children. A plan that depends on weekly direct observation may fail if no supervisor is available to provide it. A plan that requires concentration the learner currently does not have may need temporary adjustment. Feasibility is part of the design, not an afterthought.

One useful question is: **Is the recovery plan realistic for the life that actually exists?** That question does not ask whether the learner prefers the plan or whether it feels easy. It asks whether the time, energy, supervision, and logistics required are actually available. If the answer is no, the plan needs to change or the surrounding conditions need attention. A plan that cannot be executed cannot provide useful evidence about whether the learner can improve.

This is especially important after a setback because learners often respond by adding more. More study time, more meetings, more practice, and more monitoring can quickly produce a schedule that has no margin left. The plan may then collapse under its own demands. That collapse can be misread as another failure of discipline. Sometimes the better intervention is to remove something before adding more.

Temporary limitations still matter when deciding what a recovery plan can reasonably require. Illness, severe exhaustion, or another temporary reduction in capacity does not remove the standard the learner ultimately needs to meet. It may change what can realistically be demonstrated now and what conditions are needed for a useful reassessment.

Timing matters. Early in recovery, the practical question may be what the learner can reasonably execute under current conditions. Later, the question may become whether performance improves after the limiting condition changes. If it does, that provides useful evidence. If it does not, another explanation may deserve more attention. Capacity should shape the recovery plan without becoming a complete explanation for the original setback.

The Capacity-Demand Map

Take the current recovery plan and list what it requires. Include time, concentration, sleep, transportation, supervision, finances, childcare, emotional bandwidth, and any other practical demand that matters. Then compare those requirements with what is actually available in the next two weeks. The aim is not to create a perfect schedule. The aim is to identify where the plan is already depending on capacity that does not exist.

Ask four questions:

- What does this plan require from me?
- Which of those demands are realistic right now?
- Which constraints can I change?
- Which constraints require help, accommodation, or institutional action?

The map should lead to a practical adjustment. You may reduce the number of resources, move practice to a protected period, ask for clearer supervision, or address a logistical barrier that keeps interfering with the plan. In other cases, the correct response may be to seek formal accommodation or change the conditions under which the work is expected to happen. The exercise helps you see whether the plan is actually feasible.

When the System Needs to Change

Some recovery problems cannot be solved by asking the learner to become more efficient. If supervision is inadequate, someone has to improve supervision. If expectations conflict, someone has to clarify them. If the workload makes a required recovery plan impossible to complete, the workload or the plan needs reconsideration. Responsibility may therefore extend beyond the learner.

Learning-environment research gives good reason to include workload and conditions when thinking about trainee functioning (Dyrbye et al., 2009; Dyrbye et al., 2014; Dyrbye et al., 2021). Those findings do not establish that a particular environment caused a particular failed exam or clinical problem. They support the narrower point that context belongs in the analysis of what a learner can sustain. Environmental conditions can affect functioning without explaining every aspect of the original setback. Evidence still has to determine how much weight they deserve.

Recovery depends on more than knowing what to do. The learner also needs enough capacity, time, support, and structure to carry out the plan and learn from it. When those conditions are missing, the failure of the plan should not automatically be interpreted as failure of the person. The better question is what the plan requires and whether the system can actually supply it. **Recovery has infrastructure.**

Chapter 11: Recovery Is Relational

A setback changes social questions as well as academic ones. You may start wondering who knows, who needs to know, whether asking for help will make things worse, or whether people will see you differently. Those questions can make recovery feel private even when the problem requires other people. Some relationships can help you understand what happened, while others can help you act on it. The challenge is knowing who is useful for what.

How you understand and respond to a setback is shaped partly by the people around you. Belonging is a basic human motivation, and connection has been discussed as important to trainee resilience and functioning (Baumeister & Leary, 1995; McKenna et al., 2016). That does not mean relationships automatically improve recovery. Some relationships are supportive, some are neutral, and some are part of the problem. The useful question is what kind of relationship you need for the problem in front of you.

Who Knows?

After a setback, disclosure can feel risky. You may wonder whether classmates know about the failed exam, whether faculty have discussed the evaluation, or whether a remediation plan will change how people see you. You may also worry that asking for help will make the problem seem more serious. Those concerns can lead you to tell no one. Silence can feel safer when you do not yet know what the consequences are.

Secrecy usually has a function. It may protect privacy, reduce embarrassment, prevent unwanted advice, or limit exposure in an environment you do not fully trust. Sometimes the feared consequences of disclosure are larger than the actual risk. Sometimes the fear is realistic because programs differ in confidentiality, culture, and how information is used. The point is to understand what you are protecting before deciding whether disclosure helps.

More disclosure is not automatically better. A classmate may be a good source of companionship and a poor source of accurate policy information. A supervisor may be able to clarify performance expectations but may not be the person you want to process embarrassment with. A program director may have authority to make a decision but cannot promise confidentiality beyond the role. Choosing carefully can protect both privacy and usefulness.

Different People Serve Different Functions

One person rarely needs to do everything. A friend may help you feel less alone, while a faculty coach may be better at analyzing performance. An administrator may know the policy, while an advocate may be able to intervene when the process is not working fairly. A mentor may help you think about the future without having authority over the immediate decision. **Do not ask one relationship to do every job.**

It can help to think in functions. A **witness** understands what happened and takes the experience seriously. An **interpreter** helps you make sense of the event, while an **information source** gives you facts about policy, requirements, or process. A **coach** helps diagnose performance, and an **advocate** can act within the institution when action is needed. A **companion** offers steadiness without turning every conversation back toward the setback.

The same person may fill more than one role, but the distinction still matters. A close friend may be excellent at reassurance and have no idea what remediation actually means. A faculty advisor may understand the system and still be the wrong person to evaluate whether the feedback was fair. Confusion happens when you ask one relationship to provide a kind of help it cannot reliably offer. Matching the person to the function makes support more useful.

Support Is Not the Same as Reassurance

Support does not always sound comforting. A useful response may be, *We do not know yet what this means for your future, so let us figure out what is established and what information you need next.* That answer leaves uncertainty in place. It also prevents someone from promising an outcome they cannot know. Good support can help you function without pretending the uncertainty has disappeared.

Reassurance can become tempting because everyone wants the discomfort to settle. A friend may say, *You will definitely be fine,* or a mentor may insist that one setback will never matter again. Those statements may feel good and still be unsupported. If the consequences are genuinely uncertain, reassurance can replace one inaccurate story with another. Support is more useful when it stays close to what is known.

The best support does not always reduce uncertainty. Sometimes it helps you tolerate uncertainty without turning it into a conclusion about your future.

That kind of support can sound less dramatic. Someone may help you draft the email, interpret the policy, prepare questions for a meeting, or review the feedback before you decide what it means. The person does not need to make you feel better immediately. They need to help you become more able to respond. Function remains the priority.

The Relationship Around Feedback Matters

Feedback does not arrive in a vacuum. A learner may hear the same criticism differently from a supervisor who has observed them carefully and explained the concern than from someone who offered a vague judgment after limited contact. Earlier chapters asked how credible the evidence is. Here the question is whether the relationship makes the information usable. Trust and clarity affect whether the learner can engage with what is being said.

A strong feedback relationship does not require the learner to like the message. The supervisor may identify a serious problem and still explain what they observed, why it matters, and what improvement would look like. That gives the learner a path forward. A humiliating or dismissive interaction can make even accurate feedback harder to use. The quality of the relationship can therefore affect the educational value of the information.

This distinction is important because learners may otherwise conclude that difficulty accepting feedback proves defensiveness. Sometimes defensiveness is part of the problem and needs attention. Other times the learner is trying to interpret vague, inconsistent, or poorly delivered information. The useful question is what part belongs to the content and what part belongs to the relationship around it. Both can matter without being the same problem.

Connection Without Dependence

Support becomes less useful when its main job is to provide certainty. You may find yourself repeatedly asking someone, *Do you think I am going to be okay?* The answer can calm you briefly, but it may not change what you know. When uncertainty returns, you need reassurance again. The relationship starts carrying a question that no one can actually answer yet.

A more useful request is often narrower. You can ask someone to help you understand what is known, what remains uncertain, and what needs to happen next. You can ask a coach whether the same performance problem appears across settings, or ask an advisor which consequences are established by policy. Those questions give the other person something they can actually help with. They also return some control to you.

This does not mean emotional support is unimportant. There are times when you need someone who can simply acknowledge that the situation is painful and stay present without trying to solve it. That is a real function. Problems begin when companionship is expected to replace accurate information or professional guidance. Different needs deserve different relationships.

Build a Recovery Team

A useful recovery team can be small. You may need one person for steadiness, one for performance diagnosis, and one for institutional information. Another situation may require an advocate or someone with authority to make a formal decision. The exact number matters less than whether the important functions are covered. A few well-chosen relationships are usually more useful than telling everyone.

You can make the team concrete by assigning one person to each need. A friend may be the person you call after a difficult meeting, while a faculty coach reviews clinical performance. A course director may clarify remediation requirements, and a mentor may help you think about longer-term decisions. If a formal accommodation or appeal is needed, the relevant institutional office becomes part of the plan. Naming the function prevents you from asking the wrong person for the wrong kind of help.

Some problems require authority rather than support. A friend cannot approve an accommodation, and a mentor cannot always change a progression decision. If the issue involves policy, appeal, workload, mistreatment, or formal remediation, someone with institutional responsibility may need to act.

Emotional support can help you approach that process. It cannot substitute for the decision itself.

When the Relationship Is Part of the Problem

Not every relationship around a setback is safe or useful. A supervisor may be humiliating, confidentiality may feel uncertain, or a learner may believe that seeking help will increase stigma. Learners in remediation have described confidentiality as important to whether they felt able to seek support, although those findings should not be generalized to every program or trainee (Hayashi et al., 2022). Some fears about disclosure are therefore realistic. Recovery should not depend on pretending that every institutional relationship is trustworthy.

When the relationship is part of the problem, the response may need to change. You may need another supervisor, a different source of feedback, clearer boundaries, or someone who can advocate within the institution. In some cases, formal reporting or policy processes may be relevant. The point is not to force connection where the conditions make it unsafe or unhelpful. Support only works when the relationship can actually perform the function you need.

Recovery rarely happens entirely alone, but connection is useful only when it fits the problem. Some people can help you understand what happened, some can help you improve, and some can help you navigate the system. Others may simply help you stay steady while the work continues. You do not need one person who can do everything. **You need the right relationship for the job in front of you.**

A Note for Families, Partners, and Close Friends

When someone you love is facing a training setback, support usually begins with steadiness. The most useful first move is to understand what has actually happened before interpreting what it means about the person.

Try to help them separate facts, fears, deadlines, and next decisions. Practical support may matter as much as emotional support, especially when the learner is tired, ashamed, or overloaded.

Support does not require you to fix medical training from the outside. It asks you to stay close enough to listen, ask what is needed, and respect that some institutional or professional questions may take time to answer.

Part IV: Returning Without Becoming the Setback

You can be finished with remediation and still feel changed by what happened. You may have passed the repeated exam, returned to the rotation, or met the required standard while still feeling behind, marked, or uncertain about where you belong. The administrative problem may be over while the personal meaning of it remains unsettled. That does not mean recovery has failed. Performance and identity do not always recover on the same schedule.

The next questions are different from the ones that came earlier. What was actually lost, and what remains intact? What does being later really establish, and what has comparison added to the story? Can you return to a group without being reduced to the setback, and how much explanatory power should this event have in the life you build around it? These questions ask what place the setback deserves now that the immediate problem is no longer the only thing in view.

Some people will need to make substantial sense of what happened. Others may eventually regard the setback as an unpleasant period they handled and moved beyond. There is no requirement to turn disruption into a defining experience, a lesson, or a source of growth. Meaning can remain complicated, limited, or unfinished. The work is to keep the story answerable to what actually happened.

Chapter 12: The Setback May Have Taken Something

A setback can be technically resolved while something about it still hurts. You may pass the repeated exam, complete remediation, or return from leave and still feel the absence of what you expected to have. The loss may be obvious, such as time, money, or an opportunity. It may also be harder to name, such as moving forward with your cohort or trusting that effort would keep your plans intact. Naming what was lost can help explain why the experience still matters.

That loss will not look the same for everyone. Repeating a year may feel devastating to one student because close friends are graduating without them. Another student may feel relief because the original pace had become impossible to sustain. Someone else may care most about debt, geography, visa status, or a changed application timeline. **You cannot know what was lost simply by knowing what happened.**

The Visible Loss and the Invisible Loss

Administrative consequences are usually easy to describe. Graduation is delayed, an examination is repeated, a rotation must be completed again, or an application cycle changes. These facts matter because they affect what happens next. They still may not explain why the event feels so significant. The most painful loss may sit underneath the administrative one.

A delayed graduation date may also mean separation from a cohort. A leave may mean losing a role or routine that had organized daily life. A change in specialty plans may involve giving up an imagined future that had been present for years. None of those losses has to look dramatic from the outside to matter to the person experiencing it. The important question is what actually changed for you.

The answer may also surprise you. You may discover that the part you expected to miss most does not bother you much, while something smaller does. You may feel grief about one part and relief about another. You may also feel very little once the practical consequences are settled. The event does not prescribe the emotional response.

Loss Is Broader Than Bereavement

The language of loss can be useful here, but it needs a boundary. Worden's work on mourning concerns bereavement after death, so it should not be treated as evidence that an educational setback is equivalent to bereavement (Worden, 2009). The useful borrowing is narrower: people sometimes have to actively adjust to what is no longer available. That idea can help when a setback changes something the learner had reasonably expected to continue.

This does not mean you need to grieve every disrupted plan. Research on responses to loss and adversity describes substantial variation in how people respond, including trajectories that do not involve prolonged distress (Bonanno, 2004). That work should not be used to classify academic setbacks as trauma. It supports a simpler point about variation. Different people can experience the same kind of disruption very differently.

The question therefore is not *What am I supposed to feel?* The better question is what, if anything, the setback actually cost you. For one person, that answer may be time and money. For another, it may be confidence in a plan that once seemed secure. For someone else, the honest answer may be very little beyond inconvenience.

Sometimes the Loss Is an Assumption

A setback can also disturb beliefs that had quietly organized your expectations. You may have believed that hard work reliably produces success, that careful preparation gives you control, or that your career will unfold in a predictable sequence. Those beliefs may have worked well enough for years that you never had reason to examine them. A major disruption can make them suddenly visible. Losing an assumption can be disorienting even when nothing tangible has disappeared.

Janoff-Bulman's work on shattered assumptions comes from trauma research (Janoff-Bulman, 1992). The framework is useful because it draws attention to expectations that once felt stable and no longer do. An academic or professional setback is not being equated with trauma. The narrower idea is that disrupted expectations can require adjustment. Sometimes what changed was your sense of how predictable the path was.

That adjustment does not require replacing the old assumption with a cynical one. *Hard work guarantees success* may become *effort matters, and outcomes also depend on preparation, conditions, assessment, and factors I cannot fully control. If I prepare well, nothing major will go wrong* may become a more modest understanding of what preparation can and cannot guarantee. The new belief does not have to be inspiring. It only needs to fit the evidence better.

Separate Loss From Uncertainty

After a setback, feared losses can feel as real as confirmed ones. You may know that graduation is delayed and fear that residency options are permanently damaged. You may know that a supervisor raised a concern and fear that your reputation has changed everywhere. The confirmed loss and the anticipated loss can quickly blend together. Separating them makes planning more accurate.

Some consequences are already established. You may have lost time, money, an application opportunity, a position in your original cohort, or access to a particular path. Those losses deserve to be named plainly. Other consequences remain possible or unknown. **Separate what has been lost from what is still uncertain.**

This does not require you to stop worrying about uncertain outcomes. Fear can arrive long before information does. The point is to avoid planning as though every feared consequence has already occurred. You need different responses to a confirmed loss and a possible one. One may require adjustment, while the other may require information.

The Loss Inventory

Take one setback and answer the following questions in plain language.

What changed?

Name the concrete consequence.

What had I expected instead?

Describe the path, timing, opportunity, or relationship you assumed would continue.

What was actually lost?

Include tangible and less visible losses.

What remains intact?

Name what the setback did not change.

What remains uncertain?

List the consequences you fear but cannot yet establish.

The exercise is useful because setbacks tend to expand in memory. A delayed year can begin to feel like a lost career, and one closed opportunity can begin to feel like the loss of every future option. Writing down what is gone and what remains can expose where the event has grown beyond the facts. It can also reveal losses you have been minimizing because they seem less important than the academic consequence. Accuracy works in both directions.

Some Losses Stay Losses

Some consequences cannot be made better by reframing them. An extra year of tuition may create real debt, a delayed graduation may affect family plans, and a closed opportunity may remain closed. A health change may permanently alter what kind of work is possible. Calling those outcomes meaningful or beneficial can become another way of refusing to name their cost. **Accuracy sometimes means allowing a loss to remain a loss.**

You also do not need to prove that the setback made you stronger. Some experiences become important turning points, while others remain things people wish had never happened. Both possibilities fit within recovery. Integration does not require gratitude for the event. You can adapt to a loss without deciding that the loss was necessary.

This matters because medical culture often rewards polished hindsight. People tell stories in which every difficulty eventually becomes useful, and every detour appears to have led somewhere important. Real experience is usually less tidy. Some consequences lead to growth, some lead to compromise, and some simply hurt. Your account does not need a lesson before it can be accurate.

A setback may have taken something real from you. Naming that loss does not mean everything has been lost, and refusing to romanticize it does not mean recovery has failed. The task is to identify what changed, what remains, and what is still unknown. Some losses can be adapted to, while others may continue to matter for a long time. **You can let the loss be real without asking it to explain everything that comes next.**

Chapter 13: The Timeline Changed. What Does That Mean?

A changed timeline is difficult to ignore in medical training because time is always visible. Your classmates graduate, residents move up a year, applications open, and people begin jobs while you are repeating, waiting, or reapplying. The difference can be measured in months, training levels, or milestones. It can also start to feel like a ranking. *They moved forward, and I did not.*

That comparison can turn chronology into a story about competence. If someone else reached the next stage first, it is easy to assume that they are better prepared, more capable, or more suited to medicine. Sometimes a delay does reflect a performance problem that needed correction. That correction took additional time still does not make elapsed time a complete measure of ability. **A timeline difference can become a competence story even when competence and chronology are not the same variable.**

Time Matters

There is no need to pretend that timelines are meaningless. An additional semester or year can affect tuition, debt, income, insurance, visa status, application cycles, and where you are able to live. It may change caregiving arrangements, relationships, family planning, or when you can begin the next stage of training. Those consequences can be substantial. A changed timeline deserves practical planning because time has real costs.

The social cost can matter too. Your classmates may become residents while you remain a student, or your original co-residents may advance while you repeat part of a year. Shared routines and relationships can change when people who expected to progress together no longer do. You may have to enter a new cohort where everyone else already knows one another. Being later can therefore affect belonging as well as logistics.

Acknowledging those consequences is different from deciding what they mean about your ability. A delay may have happened because you had not yet demonstrated a required competency. It may have resulted from illness, leave, remediation, life circumstances, an unsuccessful application, or several factors together. The cause needs to be understood on its own evidence. **The calendar cannot do that analysis for you.**

Time and Competence Are Not the Same Measure

Medical training traditionally links progress with time. Students move through academic years, residents through postgraduate levels, and many assessments are tied to expected performance at a particular stage. That structure makes time useful for organizing training. It can also make being later feel like evidence that something is fundamentally wrong. The structure encourages a comparison that the evidence may not support.

Work on competency-based and time-variable medical education supports a narrower distinction between elapsed time and demonstrated competence (ten Cate et al., 2018). Time and competence are related within training, but they are not interchangeable measures. Taking longer to demonstrate a competency does not mean the competency no longer matters. It means the standard and the time required to reach it need to be considered separately.

This distinction should not be stretched too far. Time can provide important information, especially when difficulty persists despite appropriate teaching, practice, and support. Repeated inability to meet a standard over time may eventually become meaningful evidence about the problem. That conclusion comes from the pattern of performance, not simply from being later than someone else. Time becomes informative when we know what happened during it.

The Comparison Problem

Timeline changes become especially painful when the comparison group is close. It is one thing to know abstractly that people finish training at different ages. It is another to see the classmates you studied with begin residency while you remain behind. Their progress may appear in your messages, social media, hospital hallways, or conversations with mutual friends. The comparison is real because the difference is real.

What the comparison measures is more limited. Your classmate's graduation date tells you when they graduated, and your delayed date tells you that your path changed. Those dates do not compare every part of your knowledge, clinical ability, judgment, or future performance. They also do not tell you how either career will look several years later. A calendar can record sequence without explaining the person moving through it.

This is one reason timeline shame can persist after the original problem has been corrected. You may pass the exam or complete remediation while continuing to think of yourself as the person who is behind. Each new milestone reached by your former cohort can reactivate that comparison. The original performance problem may be finished while the chronology remains visible. Technical recovery does not automatically erase the social meaning attached to time.

Behind What?

The sentence *I am behind* sounds specific until you ask what it means. Behind whom, according to which schedule, and in what part of training? What consequence has actually occurred because of the delay? Which consequence are you predicting but cannot yet establish? Turning the statement into smaller questions makes it easier to see what requires action.

You may be one year behind your original cohort in graduation date. That can create additional tuition and delay income, which are concrete consequences. You may also fear that every future employer will see the delay as evidence that you are less capable. That conclusion requires information you do not yet have. The first problem needs planning, while the second still needs evidence.

The same distinction applies when you compare yourself with individual peers. A former classmate may now be a PGY-1 while you are completing an additional year of medical school. That difference is obvious and may be painful every time you see it. It tells you where each of you is in the sequence today. It does not provide a complete comparison of the physicians either of you will become.

When *behind* starts carrying too much meaning, make it operational. Ask who you are behind, by how much, in which domain, and with what established consequence. Then separate those facts from the conclusions you are attaching to them. The exercise does not make the delay disappear. It makes the problem specific enough to plan around.

The Timeline Does Not Need to Become Inspirational

A changed timeline does not have to become a lesson about how everyone moves at their own pace. That message can feel dismissive when an extra year has created debt, disrupted relationships, or closed an opportunity. You are allowed to prefer the original timeline. You are also allowed to acknowledge that the change created consequences you would have chosen to avoid.

You do not need to turn the delay into evidence that everything happens for a reason. Some delays later become meaningful, while others remain frustrating or costly parts of a career. The future may contain benefits you cannot currently predict, but there is no need to invent them now. Accuracy does not require optimism. It requires giving the timeline the meaning the evidence supports.

A more useful statement is simpler. **This is not the timeline you wanted, and it may have consequences.** Those consequences deserve planning, whether they involve money, applications, relationships, or additional training. They deserve the same specificity used elsewhere in this book. **They do not automatically answer what physician you can become.**

A Timeline Check

When the thought *I am behind* appears, write down what you mean. Identify the person or schedule you are comparing yourself with, the amount of time involved, and the concrete consequence of the difference. Then list any future consequence you are assuming but cannot yet establish. This separates chronology from the conclusions that have gathered around it.

Ask five questions:

- Behind whom?
- According to which expected schedule?
- In what specific domain?
- What consequence has actually occurred?
- What consequence am I predicting?

The answers may still be difficult. You may discover costs that require real changes in finances, applications, geography, or family plans. You may also discover that some of what felt like fact was comparison or prediction. Both pieces matter because they require different responses. A precise timeline is easier to plan around than the global feeling of being behind.

A changed timeline is real, and the cost of it may also be real. Being later can affect money, relationships, opportunities, and how you experience your place among peers. What it does not do automatically is measure everything that matters about your professional ability. The delay deserves to be understood for what it actually changed. **A timeline can matter without measuring everything that matters about you.**

Chapter 14: Returning to the Room

You can return to training before you feel as though you are fully back. The schedule may show that remediation is complete, your badge may work again, and you may be standing in the same hallway with everyone else. None of that guarantees that the room feels the same. You may wonder who knows, what people have heard, or whether every mistake will now be noticed differently. Administrative return and social return are not always the same thing.

That distinction matters because belonging in medicine is partly social. Professional identity develops through participation, recognition, role models, institutional culture, and interaction with other people in training (Monrouxe, 2010; Cruess et al., 2014; Cruess et al., 2015). A recent theoretical review also examines identity struggles within medical training directly (Sawatsky et al., 2026). Returning therefore involves more than resuming tasks. **Belonging is also about whether the environment still allows you to participate as someone who can keep developing.**

You May Feel Marked

A learner can finish remediation and still feel as though the label remains. You may walk into rounds wondering whether the attending already knows, or sit beside classmates wondering what was said while you were away. A correction that was educational on paper can begin to feel social once it changes how you imagine other people see you. The concern may be subtle, but it can shape how much you speak, ask for help, or take ordinary risks in learning. Returning can become an exercise in watching yourself.

Sometimes that feeling is based mainly on uncertainty. Almost nobody may know what happened, and the people around you may be thinking far less about it than you imagine. In other situations, the setback is genuinely visible because you changed cohorts, repeated a rotation, or entered a formal remediation process. The difference matters because the response should fit the reality. *Everyone knows* can be an anxious inference or an accurate description of the situation.

Visibility itself is not the whole problem. The harder issue is what other people conclude from what they know. A repeated exam may be visible without explaining the learner's current competence. A remediation plan may be known without establishing how the learner will perform six months later. The social risk begins when an educational event becomes a fixed identity. A temporary intervention should not automatically become a permanent description.

Disclosure Is Not All or Nothing

After a setback, disclosure can feel like a moral question when it is really a practical one. You may wonder whether hiding what happened means you are ashamed, or whether telling people is necessary to prove that you have accepted it. Neither conclusion is required. Privacy can be reasonable, especially when the information is personal or professionally sensitive. **Privacy is not the same as shame-driven secrecy.**

It helps to distinguish different kinds of disclosure. Some information is **required** because a program, supervisor, licensing body, or other authority legitimately needs it. Some disclosure is **useful** because another person can help with support, planning, or advocacy. Other disclosure is **optional** because the information belongs to you and serves no necessary function. In some settings, disclosure may also be unwise if the relationship is unsafe or the information is likely to be misused.

The useful question is what the disclosure is for. Telling a trusted friend may provide steadiness, while telling a supervisor may clarify expectations or allow the right support to be arranged. Telling a casual acquaintance may add exposure without adding anything useful. More disclosure does not automatically produce more recovery. The amount of disclosure should match the function it serves.

Returning Under Observation

Some learners return to training knowing that observation has increased. A remediation plan may require direct supervision, repeated assessments, or closer review over a defined period. In that setting, telling the learner to stop worrying about what people think misses the reality of the situation. More people may genuinely be watching performance because the program needs evidence that the problem has been corrected. The better response is to make the observation transparent.

A learner should know what successful reintegration requires. Which behaviors or competencies are being assessed, who will observe them, and over what period of time? What counts as sufficient improvement, and what happens when the criteria are met? Unclear observation can make every interaction feel consequential. Clear criteria turn increased scrutiny back into an educational process.

This matters because self-monitoring can otherwise become constant. One awkward presentation may feel like proof that remediation has failed, and one supervisor's neutral expression may become evidence that the label remains. Transparent criteria reduce the need to interpret every small cue. The learner can focus on the behaviors that actually count. Re-entry becomes easier when success is something that can be demonstrated rather than guessed at.

Re-entry and Reintegration

Re-entry answers an administrative question. Are you back in the course, rotation, program, or role? Reintegration asks whether you can participate again without being continually reduced to what happened. Those processes can move at different speeds. A learner may be formally returned while still feeling socially separate.

Performance can recover on yet another timeline. You may meet the required standard before you trust your own performance again. You may also feel socially comfortable before the program has collected enough evidence to remove additional supervision. These differences do not mean something has gone wrong. They show that administrative status, performance, relationships, and belonging are separate parts of return.

The Reintegration Map

A simple map can help clarify where the remaining problem sits:

- **Administrative:** Am I formally back?
- **Performance:** Have I demonstrated the required standard?
- **Relational:** Can I work with supervisors and peers without the setback dominating the interaction?
- **Belonging:** Do I experience myself as a participant again?

The categories do not need to recover together. You may be doing well clinically while still feeling like an outsider, or you may feel welcomed socially while waiting for a formal progression decision. Knowing which part is unfinished prevents one problem from being mistaken for all of them. It also makes the next step easier to identify. Reintegration becomes more manageable when you know what kind of return is still missing.

The Environment Has Responsibilities Too

A learner cannot complete reintegration alone. The learner can meet expectations, respond to feedback, demonstrate competence, and produce new evidence. The institution also has to be willing to update its interpretation when that evidence changes. If successful performance never alters how the learner is viewed, remediation has stopped functioning as a developmental process. A pathway back requires the possibility of being seen differently.

This is where fairness becomes practical. Accountability requires learners to respond to new evidence about their performance. Fairness requires institutions to respond to new evidence about the learner. A concern that was justified six months ago should not be treated as permanently current if subsequent performance no longer supports it. **A learner cannot fully reintegrate into an environment that refuses to update its interpretation of them.**

Successful remediation should therefore have an endpoint that means something. If the learner meets the stated criteria, there should be a genuine pathway out of the label rather than indefinite suspicion. Treating remediation as part of training is consistent with the idea that difficulty can be identified, addressed, and reassessed rather than converted into a permanent mark against the person (Kalet et al., 2017). Without that possibility, the learner carries an educational event as an ongoing social sentence. Reintegration depends on the institution recognizing when the evidence has changed.

What If People Do See You Differently?

Some relationships may change after a visible setback. A supervisor may watch more closely, a peer may ask questions, or a new cohort may know that you joined them after repeating part of training. You cannot control every interpretation other people make. You can control whether your own attention stays anchored to the evidence that matters. The goal is participation, not management of every possible opinion.

That may mean asking for clear expectations instead of trying to read the room. It may mean deciding in advance what you will disclose and to whom. It may also mean noticing when you are treating every ordinary mistake as proof that the label has returned. The more transparent the standards are, the less work you have to spend guessing how you are being judged. Reintegration becomes more possible when the criteria for success are visible.

Returning to the room can be administratively simple and socially complicated. You may be back before you feel back, and other people may need time and evidence to update how they see you. What matters is whether participation remains possible and whether the standards for successful return are clear. Reintegration does not require pretending the setback never happened. It requires allowing what happens next to count.

Chapter 15: What Story Will This Become?

A setback can begin as one event and later become the explanation for everything that came before it. You fail an exam, then remember every course that ever felt difficult. You receive a concerning evaluation, then reinterpret years of uncertainty as evidence that the problem had always been there. The event starts organizing memories that once had different meanings. A story begins to form around it.

That process matters because identity is shaped partly through the stories people tell about their lives and how they connect events across time (McAdams, 2001). A setback may therefore become part of how a learner understands their training, competence, and future. The problem begins when one event is given more explanatory power than the evidence supports. **A difficult chapter can become the plot of the entire book when one event is asked to explain too much.**

The Setback Can Become the Organizing Plot

Imagine a student who struggled in anatomy, performed well during clinical rotations, and has always found standardized tests difficult. After failing one major examination, those separate facts may be reorganized into a new story. *I have always been someone who cannot handle medicine.* The failure now explains anatomy, testing, previous uncertainty, and fears about the future. A single event has turned several different experiences into one conclusion.

The new story may feel more coherent than the old one. Before the failure, the student had a mixed record with strengths, weaknesses, and unresolved questions. Afterward, the record seems to point in one direction. Coherence can feel convincing because it removes ambiguity. It can still be inaccurate if important evidence has been left out.

This is the same process in a later form. A setback first becomes a conclusion about competence or belonging. Over time, that conclusion can become a story about who you have always been. Earlier events are then reread through the new story. The past starts looking inevitable.

Meaning Does Not Have to Arrive Quickly

There is often pressure to decide what a major disruption means. You may feel that you should know whether the setback changed you, taught you something, or redirected your career. Other people may ask what you learned from it before you have finished dealing with the consequences. The question can feel premature when the event is still unfolding. Some meanings become clearer only with distance.

You do not owe the setback its final meaning while you are still inside it.

A significant setback may enter your developing self-story even if you never sit down to reflect deliberately on it. You may notice yourself referring to life as *before I failed* and *after I failed,* or interpreting later experiences through what happened during remediation. That does not mean the event must become central forever. Stories can change when new evidence arrives.

The story can also remain unfinished. You may understand what happened educationally and still be unsure what it means personally. You may know that the setback changed your timeline without knowing whether it changed the physician you will become. Uncertainty is a legitimate position. Meaning does not become more accurate simply because it is complete.

Narrative Reconstruction Is Not Positive Thinking

Revising the story does not mean finding a more positive version of it. *This ruined everything* may stretch the evidence, while *this was the best thing that ever happened to me* can distort it in the opposite direction. The aim is not to replace a painful story with an inspiring one. The aim is to make the account more accurate. Accuracy may still include disappointment, anger, loss, or regret.

A realistic narrative can contain mistakes and external failures at the same time. You may have prepared poorly while also receiving inadequate guidance. You may have needed remediation while also being treated unfairly during part of the process. You may have grown from correcting a weakness while still wishing the setback had never happened. A coherent story does not require removing complexity.

That matters because polished hindsight is common in medicine. Career stories often make the past look purposeful, as though each difficulty was necessary for what came next. Real training is usually messier. Some experiences teach something useful, while others simply cost time, money, confidence, or opportunity. Your story does not need to justify what happened.

Separate the Event From the Explanation

A story becomes more accurate when you separate what happened from what you have made it explain. The event may be *I failed the examination*. The explanation might be *my study strategy was poorly matched to the exam and I had important knowledge gaps*. The broader story might become *I have always lacked the ability to succeed in medicine*. Those statements do not carry the same evidentiary weight. The last one needs much more support than the first two.

This separation can reveal how much work one event has been asked to do. A learner who failed an exam may start using the failure to explain earlier insecurity, present difficulty, and every feared future outcome. The event becomes evidence about intelligence, belonging, work ethic, and career potential all at once. That is an enormous amount of explanatory responsibility for one result. **The story remains answerable to the evidence.**

One way to test the story is to ask what evidence it leaves out. If the story says *I have always been bad clinically,* what do previous evaluations show? If it says *I never belonged here,* what evidence existed before the setback that supported the opposite conclusion? If it says *this ruined my career,* which consequences are established and which remain uncertain? A story becomes more accurate when contrary evidence is allowed back in.

Watch for Narrative Absolutes

Certain words can signal that the story has become larger than the evidence. *Always, never, everyone, ruined, finally,* and *proved* are worth slowing down around. They may still be accurate in a particular sentence. More often, they compress a complicated record into a complete conclusion. The word itself is not the problem. The question is whether the evidence can support its size.

Consider the sentence *I have always struggled academically*. That may feel true immediately after a failure. A closer review may show strong performance in most courses, difficulty with standardized exams, and one subject that required unusual effort. The narrower description may still identify a real weakness. It simply stops one weakness from describing everything.

The same applies to social conclusions. *Everyone knows* may mean three classmates know because your cohort changed. *My supervisors will never trust me again* may reflect fear before enough time has passed to know how they will respond to new performance. Converting absolutes into specific statements does not make the story more positive. It makes it easier to check.

You Are Allowed to Keep the Complicated Version

Some setbacks never resolve into one clean meaning. You may believe the event exposed a real weakness while also believing the institution handled it badly. You may appreciate skills you developed during remediation while still resenting the cost. You may feel proud of how you responded and embarrassed that the event happened at all. None of those tensions need to be eliminated for the story to be coherent.

A complicated story can be more accurate than a polished one. It allows the learner, the environment, chance, timing, and changing circumstances to have separate roles. It also leaves room for later evidence to change the interpretation again. You do not have to decide which single explanation deserves ownership of the whole experience. A complicated account is appropriate when the experience itself was complicated.

This matters when other people ask for a simplified account. Applications, interviews, advising conversations, and casual questions may all encourage a clean narrative. You can give a concise answer for a specific purpose without making that answer your entire private understanding of the event. A useful public account and a complete personal account are not always the same thing. Your story can remain more complicated than the version a situation requires.

Narrative Medicine as a Lens

Narrative medicine offers useful questions about how stories are constructed, although it does not provide direct evidence about recovery from academic setbacks (Charon, 2006). The value here is methodological. A story can be examined for what it includes, what it omits, which events it links causally, and where it places agency. Those questions help reveal when hindsight has made one interpretation seem inevitable.

Ask what your current story emphasizes. Does it include only the failure and exclude the years of competence before it? Does it make the setback the cause of difficulties that began for unrelated reasons? Does it describe you as passive in places where you made choices, or entirely responsible where the environment also mattered? Examining the structure of the story can make hidden assumptions visible.

The point is not to become your own literary critic. It is to notice when the way the story is organized has started influencing what you believe about yourself. A different organization may fit the evidence better. The underlying facts do not need to change. Their relationship to one another might.

The Three Versions Exercise

Write three short versions of the setback. Each version should be brief enough to read in less than a minute. The purpose is to notice how the same event changes depending on what you ask it to explain. Do not try to make the third version inspiring. It only needs to be more accurate.

The threat story

Write the version that appeared when the setback felt most threatening. Include the fears, assumptions, and conclusions that came with it.

The administrative story

Write only what happened in concrete terms. Include the failed assessment, evaluation, remediation, delay, leave, or other established consequence.

The current working story

Write what you now believe based on the evidence you have. Include what went wrong, what contributed, what changed, what remains uncertain, and what you no longer think the event can establish.

The third version may still be painful. It may say that you had a serious knowledge deficit, that your timeline changed, and that you lost an opportunity you wanted. It may also say that the deficit was corrected and that several feared consequences never occurred. The point is not to produce a better-feeling story. **The third version only needs to be more accurate than the first.**

Sometimes the Story Should Get Smaller

There is another possibility that deserves explicit permission. The setback may eventually stop being very important to how you understand yourself. You may fail an examination, identify several problems, correct them, pass, and move on. Years later, the event may remain memorable without carrying much meaning. That outcome does not represent failed reflection.

Meaning-making can sometimes involve reducing meaning. An event that once seemed to explain your entire future may eventually become one piece of information from one period of training. It can lose importance because later experience gives you much more evidence about who you are and what you can do. The setback does not have to remain central simply because it once felt central. **Meaning-making sometimes means reducing meaning.**

This kind of narrative minimalism can be especially useful in a culture that encourages people to extract lessons from every difficulty. Some experiences deserve reflection, while others become less important with time. You do not have to keep returning to the setback simply because it was once painful. Moving on can be an accurate response. The event can become ordinary history.

A setback may become part of the story you tell about becoming a physician. It does not need to become the explanation for everything that came before or everything that happens next. The story can remain complicated, change over time, or eventually become much smaller. New evidence deserves the chance to revise old conclusions. **The event can stay in the story without becoming the story.**

Chapter 16: Recovery Is Part of Professional Formation

Professional formation is often described through progress. You learn more, take on greater responsibility, become more independent, and gradually begin to think and act like a physician. Setbacks interrupt that picture because they introduce error, limitation, uncertainty, and sometimes a change in direction. It can be tempting to solve that discomfort by saying that failure makes better doctors. That claim asks too much of the setback.

Some setbacks are preventable, some are harmful, and some expose problems that should have been addressed earlier. Others arise partly from illness, life circumstances, poor supervision, unclear expectations, or institutional failures. A learner may recover from the event without ever believing that it was necessary or beneficial. Professional growth does not require gratitude for what happened. It requires an accurate response to what happened.

Formation Includes How You Respond to Difficulty

Becoming a physician involves more than accumulating successful performances. Training also asks you to recognize what you do not know, respond to feedback, revise decisions, seek help, and work within systems that are often imperfect. Those capacities become especially visible when something has gone wrong. A setback does not automatically produce them. Responding to the setback can require them.

Professional identity formation has been described as a process involving participation, socialization, relationships, and increasing identification with the role of physician (Cruess et al., 2014; Cruess et al., 2015). That process does not happen only during moments of success. A learner who has to examine a mistake, tolerate uncertainty, or change an ineffective approach is still participating in professional development. The difficult event is not what makes the development valuable. What matters is how accurately the learner and the surrounding system respond to it.

This distinction protects against romanticizing failure. A serious mistake does not become good because the learner eventually improves. Poor supervision does not become acceptable because the learner later develops resilience. An unnecessary delay does not become worthwhile because something was learned during it. Growth can occur after harm without making the harm desirable.

Recovery Uses Professional Capacities

Many of the skills needed for recovery are familiar professional capacities. You may need epistemic humility to admit that your first explanation was wrong, diagnostic reasoning to identify what actually caused the problem, and feedback literacy to decide which information deserves weight. You may need help-seeking, systems awareness, adaptation, and the ability to function while uncertainty remains. These are recognizable parts of professional life. Recovery brings them into unusually personal territory.

Consider what happens when a resident receives repeated feedback about clinical reasoning. The resident has to decide whether the feedback is credible, identify the specific problem, seek observation, change the approach, and review whether performance improves. Those are many of the same habits expected when physicians respond to uncertainty in clinical care. The subject is different because the learner is now part of the problem being examined. That makes the reasoning harder, not less professional.

Accountability belongs here as well. A learner may need to acknowledge that preparation was inadequate, that communication caused a problem, or that a standard has not yet been met. The professional response is to name the issue closely enough that correction becomes possible. Shame adds a judgment about the person without improving that work. Accurate accountability is a professional capacity because it keeps responsibility connected to action.

Systems awareness is equally important. Physicians are expected to understand that outcomes emerge from individuals working inside teams, workflows, institutions, and constraints. The same reasoning should apply when the learner is the person whose performance is under review. Some problems will be mainly learner problems, while others involve supervision, workload, unclear expectations, or interaction between learner and environment. Professional maturity includes being able to examine both without using either one to erase the other.

Do Not Turn Recovery Into Another Standard to Fail

There is a risk in describing recovery as part of professional formation. A learner who has already struggled can hear a new demand: now I also have to recover correctly. You may begin measuring whether you are reflective enough, resilient enough, sufficiently self-aware, or grateful for what you learned. Recovery becomes one more performance being observed. That is not the intention.

People respond to disruption in different ways and on different timelines. Research on responses to adversity has emphasized heterogeneity rather than one required pattern of recovery (Bonanno, 2004). That work does not establish a single model for educational setbacks. It supports the narrower point that people do not need to follow the same emotional course. **The**

professional requirement is not a particular emotional journey.

You may remain angry about what happened while still responding responsibly. You may feel embarrassed long after your performance has improved, or feel relatively little once the practical problem is solved. You may find the experience meaningful, or you may eventually stop thinking about it very much. None of those responses determines whether you have met the professional standard. The relevant question is whether you can act responsibly in relation to what occurred.

This also means that reflection has limits. Repeatedly analyzing the event does not automatically produce greater maturity. At some point, additional reflection may stop generating information and become another way of remaining inside the setback. A learner who has understood the problem, made the required changes, and demonstrated improvement may not need a deeper lesson. Sometimes moving forward is enough.

Recovery Does Not Guarantee the Original Destination

Recovery is often imagined as returning to the path you were on before something went wrong. Sometimes that is exactly what happens. You remediate an exam, complete the required work, and continue toward the same specialty and career you had planned. Other setbacks change the available options or change what you want. Recovery may therefore involve continuing differently.

A learner may change specialty after discovering that an earlier plan no longer fits. Another may transfer programs, take leave, extend training, or choose a different kind of work. Some people may eventually decide to leave medicine. These outcomes should not automatically be described as failure to recover. **Recovery is not loyalty to the old trajectory.**

That principle matters because the original plan can become another standard against which every later choice is judged. If the only acceptable ending is returning exactly to where you expected to be, any changed direction may feel like defeat. Sometimes the evidence supports staying the course, and sometimes it supports a different decision. The quality of the decision depends on how well it fits the person and the evidence available now. The earlier plan does not deserve permanent authority simply because it came first.

A changed destination may still involve loss. You may have wanted a specialty that is no longer realistic, or a particular timeline may have become impossible. Accepting that change does not require pretending you never wanted the original path. Recovery can include disappointment and redirection at the same time. A new direction becomes meaningful because it fits the present evidence, not because the old one had to fail.

The Final Accounting

At the beginning of this book, the task was to slow down what happened after a setback. An event could quickly become an explanation of ability, belonging, or the future before enough information was available. The work since then has been to separate those questions, locate the problem, test explanations, restore functioning, and decide what meaning the event deserves. Recovery becomes easier to understand when each part is accounted for separately. The final question is what actually changed.

One part of the accounting belongs to the learner. Maybe you changed how you study, ask for feedback, organize clinical work, or respond when you do not understand something. You may have learned to seek help earlier or to recognize when effort is being spent on the wrong problem. You may also have encountered a limitation that needs to remain part of future planning. Those changes should be named without turning them into a story of redemption.

Another part belongs to the environment. Supervision may have improved, expectations may have become clearer, workload may have changed, or an accommodation may finally have been put in place. An institution may also have failed to make changes that the evidence supported. The learner's improvement does not erase those failures. Recovery can occur even when the surrounding system remains imperfect.

The uncomfortable case is when both needed to change and only one did. A learner may correct a real performance problem while the institution continues to provide poor supervision. An environment may become more supportive while the learner continues avoiding feedback or failing to meet a clear standard. Those situations are harder because responsibility remains unevenly addressed. Accurate recovery requires seeing what changed and what did not.

Maturity is not deciding whose fault everything was. It is locating responsibility accurately enough that the right things can change.

What the Learner Changed and What the Environment Changed

A final review can help keep responsibility specific. Take the original setback and write down what the evidence eventually showed about your own contribution. Then identify what you actually changed in response and what evidence suggests that the change mattered. Keep the description behavioral and concrete. The aim is to see what recovery required from you.

Next, do the same for the environment. Identify what conditions contributed, what changed around you, and what remained outside your control. Include supervision, workload, expectations, policy, accommodations, or other factors that genuinely affected the situation. Do not add environmental explanations simply to make the story feel fairer. Include only what the evidence supports.

Then look at the interaction between the two. A new study strategy may have worked only after your schedule became manageable. Better supervision may have helped reveal a clinical skill gap that you then addressed. An accommodation may have increased your capacity while leaving a separate competence problem that still required practice. Recovery often becomes clearer when the interaction is visible.

Finally, name what remains unresolved. You may still disagree with part of the institutional response, remain uncertain about what caused one aspect of the setback, or carry consequences that cannot be corrected. An accurate final accounting does not need to tie every loose end. It needs to distinguish what changed from what remains unfinished.

The Physician You Become Does Not Need a Perfect Origin Story

Medicine often rewards coherent stories about becoming a physician. People describe always knowing what they wanted, learning from every challenge, and arriving at the present through a sequence that makes sense in retrospect. Those stories can be meaningful. They can also make ordinary detours, mistakes, and uncertainty feel like evidence that something has gone wrong. Real professional formation is often less tidy.

Your history may include a failed examination, a delayed year, a period of poor functioning, a difficult relationship with a supervisor, or an ambition that changed. It may include choices you regret and circumstances you could not control. Some parts may eventually make sense, while others remain unresolved. None of that requires you to create a cleaner history than the one you actually lived. Professional identity can contain complexity.

You may also find that the setback becomes less important with time. New patients, supervisors, decisions, successes, and mistakes will add more evidence about how you practice. An event that once seemed to explain everything may become one piece of a much larger record. That is a legitimate form of integration. The setback does not need permanent prominence simply because it once had it.

A different learner may continue to regard the event as important years later. It may change how they supervise others, how quickly they ask for help, or what they notice when someone else is struggling. That meaning can be real without requiring the learner to describe the original event as beneficial. Integration and gratitude are different things. **The setback does not need to become beneficial in order to become integrated.**

Recovery does not require a perfect ending. You may continue on the same path, choose another one, accept a lasting limitation, or decide that the setback deserves very little space in the story you carry forward. What matters is that the response became more accurate than the first explanation and more useful than self-condemnation. The event can become part of professional formation without becoming the reason you became a physician. **The physician you become does not need a perfect origin story.**

Conclusion

By the time you reach the end of a setback, the questions are usually different from the ones you started with. The first questions may have been about whether you still belonged, whether the future had changed, or whether the event exposed something fundamental about you. Over time, those questions can become more specific. Where did the problem actually live, what did the evidence show, and what needed to change? Recovery becomes clearer when the questions get smaller.

Some of the answers may be uncomfortable. You may discover a knowledge gap, a pattern you had been avoiding, a mistake that required accountability, or a limitation that changed what was possible. You may also discover that workload, supervision, unclear expectations, health, or circumstances around the setback mattered more than you first realized. In many cases, the final explanation will include more than one contributor. The point was never to protect you from difficult information.

It was to make the information accurate enough to use. A learner problem should be named closely enough that it can be corrected. An environmental problem should be located clearly enough that responsibility does not fall entirely on the person who received the result. A consequence should be taken seriously without being allowed to explain more than it can support. Precision makes responsibility more useful.

You may also have changed during the process. Perhaps you study differently, ask for feedback earlier, tolerate uncertainty better, or recognize sooner when you are trying to solve the wrong problem. You may have become more willing to seek help or more careful about which advice deserves weight. Some changes may be less satisfying, such as accepting a delayed timeline or a path you did not originally choose. Recovery does not require every change to feel like growth.

The environment may have changed too. Supervision may have improved, expectations may have become clearer, or an accommodation may finally have been put in place. In other situations, the environment may have changed very little, leaving you to work around a problem the institution never fully addressed. That belongs in the final accounting as much as the work you did yourself. Responsibility should remain where the evidence places it.

There may still be parts of the story you cannot settle. You may never know exactly how much one factor contributed, whether another outcome would have occurred under different conditions, or how much the setback will matter years from now. Some uncertainty survives good analysis. That does not make the work incomplete. It means the available evidence cannot answer every question about the event.

You do not need to minimize what happened. A failed exam can matter, a lost year can carry real costs, and difficult feedback can expose something that genuinely needed correction. You also do not need to turn the experience into inspiration or argue that it happened for a reason. A painful event can remain painful without controlling the rest of the story. **Accuracy does not require redemption.**

The same principle applies to identity. You do not need to erase the setback from your history, and you do not need to make it the central explanation for who you became. Later experiences will add more evidence about your competence, judgment, relationships, and ability to practice. The event may become important, ordinary, complicated, or surprisingly small with time. Its place in the story can change as the evidence changes.

The sequence remains simple:

Event before conclusion. Locate before you label. Diagnose before you redesign.

Start with what happened. Find out where the problem lives, gather enough evidence to understand it, and change what the evidence shows needs changing. Then allow what happens next to count. A setback should remain answerable to new information.

The setback is part of the story. It does not get to write the rest of it alone.

REFERENCES

Audétat, M.-C., Laurin, S., Sanche, G., Béïque, C., Caire Fon, N., Blais, J.-G., & Charlin, B. (2013). Clinical reasoning difficulties: A taxonomy for clinical teachers. *Medical Teacher, 35*(3), e984--e989. https://doi.org/10.3109/0142159X.2012.733041

Baumeister, R. F., & Leary, M. R. (1995). The need to belong: Desire for interpersonal attachments as a fundamental human motivation. *Psychological Bulletin, 117*(3), 497--529. https://doi.org/10.1037/0033-2909.117.3.497

Boileau, E., St-Onge, C., & Audétat, M.-C. (2017). Is there a way for clinical teachers to assist struggling learners? A synthetic review of the literature. *Advances in Medical Education and Practice, 8*, 89--97. https://doi.org/10.2147/AMEP.S123410

Bonanno, G. A. (2004). Loss, trauma, and human resilience: Have we underestimated the human capacity to thrive after extremely aversive events? *American Psychologist, 59*(1), 20--28. https://doi.org/10.1037/0003-066X.59.1.20

Breines, J. G., & Chen, S. (2012). Self-compassion increases self-improvement motivation. *Personality and Social Psychology Bulletin, 38*(9), 1133--1143. https://doi.org/10.1177/0146167212445599

Bynum, W. E., IV, & Goodie, J. L. (2014). Shame, guilt, and the medical learner: Ignored connections and why we should care. *Medical Education, 48*(11), 1045--1054. https://doi.org/10.1111/medu.12521

Bynum, W. E., IV, Artino, A. R., Jr., Uijtdehaage, S., Webb, A. M. B., & Varpio, L. (2019). Sentinel emotional events: The nature, triggers, and effects of shame experiences in medical residents. *Academic Medicine, 94*(1), 85--93. https://doi.org/10.1097/ACM.0000000000002479

Bynum, W. E., IV, Teunissen, P. W., & Varpio, L. (2021a). In the "shadow of shame": A phenomenological exploration of the nature of shame experiences in medical students. *Academic Medicine, 96*(11S), S23--S30. https://doi.org/10.1097/ACM.0000000000004261

Bynum, W. E., IV, Varpio, L., Lagoo, J., & Teunissen, P. W. (2021b). "I'm unworthy of being in this space": The origins of shame in medical students. *Medical Education, 55*(2), 185--197. https://doi.org/10.1111/medu.14354

Charon, R. (2006). *Narrative medicine: Honoring the stories of illness.* Oxford University Press.

Chou, C. L., Kalet, A., Costa, M. J., Cleland, J., & Winston, K. (2019). Guidelines: The dos, don'ts and don't knows of remediation in medical education. *Perspectives on Medical Education, 8*(6), 322--338. https://doi.org/10.1007/s40037-019-00544-5

Cruess, R. L., Cruess, S. R., Boudreau, J. D., Snell, L., & Steinert, Y. (2014). Reframing medical education to support professional identity formation. *Academic Medicine, 89*(11), 1446--1451. https://doi.org/10.1097/ACM.0000000000000427

Cruess, R. L., Cruess, S. R., Boudreau, J. D., Snell, L., & Steinert, Y. (2015). A schematic representation of the professional identity formation and socialization of medical students and residents: A guide for medical educators. *Academic Medicine, 90*(6), 718--725. https://doi.org/10.1097/ACM.0000000000000700

Dyrbye, L. N., Satele, D., & West, C. P. (2021). Association of characteristics of the learning environment and US medical student burnout, empathy, and career regret. *JAMA Network Open, 4*(8), e2119110. https://doi.org/10.1001/jamanetworkopen.2021.19110

Dyrbye, L. N., Thomas, M. R., Harper, W., Massie, F. S., Jr., Power, D. V., Eacker, A., Szydlo, D. W., Novotny, P. J., Sloan, J. A., & Shanafelt, T. D. (2009). The learning environment and medical student burnout: A multicentre study. *Medical Education, 43*(3), 274--282. https://doi.org/10.1111/j.1365-2923.2008.03282.x

Dyrbye, L. N., West, C. P., Satele, D., Boone, S., Tan, L., Sloan, J., & Shanafelt, T. D. (2014). Burnout among U.S. medical students, residents, and early career physicians relative to the general U.S. population. *Academic Medicine, 89*(3), 443--451. https://doi.org/10.1097/ACM.0000000000000134

Eysenck, M. W., Derakshan, N., Santos, R., & Calvo, M. G. (2007). Anxiety and cognitive performance: Attentional control theory. *Emotion, 7*(2), 336--353. https://doi.org/10.1037/1528-3542.7.2.336

Govaerts, M. J. B., van de Wiel, M. W. J., Schuwirth, L. W. T., van der Vleuten, C. P. M., & Muijtjens, A. M. M. (2013). Workplace-based assessment: Raters' performance theories and constructs. *Advances in Health Sciences Education, 18*(3), 375--396. https://doi.org/10.1007/s10459-012-9376-x

Guerrasio, J., Garrity, M. J., & Aagaard, E. M. (2014). Learner deficits and academic outcomes of medical students, residents, fellows, and attending physicians referred to a remediation program, 2006--2012. *Academic Medicine, 89*(2), 352--358. https://doi.org/10.1097/ACM.0000000000000122

Han, P. K. J., Schaufel, M., & Schei, E. (2026). Shame among medical learners: An uncertainty-focused conception. *Patient Education and Counseling, 147*, Article 109516. https://doi.org/10.1016/j.pec.2026.109516

Hauer, K. E., Park, Y. S., Bullock, J. L., & Tekian, A. (2023). "My assessments are biased!" Measurement and sociocultural approaches to achieve fairness in assessment in medical education. *Academic Medicine, 98*(8S), S16--S27. https://doi.org/10.1097/ACM.0000000000005245

Hayashi, M., Karouji, Y., & Nishiya, K. (2022). Ambivalent professional identity of early remedial medical students from Generation Z: A qualitative study. *BMC Medical Education, 22*, 501. https://doi.org/10.1186/s12909-022-03583-5

Higgins, E. T. (1987). Self-discrepancy: A theory relating self and affect. *Psychological Review, 94*(3), 319--340. https://doi.org/10.1037/0033-295X.94.3.319

Ismaeel, R., Pusic, L., Gottlieb, M., Chan, T. M., Oyedokun, T. O., & Thoma, B. (2024). Bias in observed assessments in medical education: A scoping review. *Academic Medicine, 99*(12), 1438--1450. https://doi.org/10.1097/ACM.0000000000005794

Janoff-Bulman, R. (1992). *Shattered assumptions: Towards a new psychology of trauma.* Free Press.

Kalet, A., Chou, C. L., & Ellaway, R. H. (2017). To fail is human: Remediating remediation in medical education. *Perspectives on Medical Education, 6*(6), 418--424. https://doi.org/10.1007/s40037-017-0385-6

Kalet, A., Guerrasio, J., & Chou, C. L. (2016). Twelve tips for developing and maintaining a remediation program in medical education. *Medical Teacher, 38*(8), 787--792. https://doi.org/10.3109/0142159X.2016.1150983

Kirtchuk, D., Wells, G., Levett, T., Castledine, C., & de Visser, R. (2022). Understanding the impact of academic difficulties among medical students: A scoping review. *Medical Education, 56*(3), 262--269. https://doi.org/10.1111/medu.14624

Lacasse, M., Audétat, M.-C., Boileau, É., Caire Fon, N., Dufour, M.-H., Laferrière, M.-C., Lafleur, A., La Rue, È., Lee, S., Nendaz, M., Paquette Raynard, E., Simard, C., Steinert, Y., & Théorêt, J. (2019). Interventions for undergraduate and postgraduate medical learners with academic difficulties: A BEME systematic review: BEME Guide No. 56. *Medical Teacher, 41*(9), 981--1001. https://doi.org/10.1080/0142159X.2019.1596239

LeBlanc, V. R. (2009). The effects of acute stress on performance: Implications for health professions education. *Academic Medicine, 84*(10 Suppl), S25--S33. https://doi.org/10.1097/ACM.0b013e3181b37b8f

McAdams, D. P. (2001). The psychology of life stories. *Review of General Psychology, 5*(2), 100--122. https://doi.org/10.1037/1089-2680.5.2.100

McEwen, B. S. (1998). Stress, adaptation, and disease: Allostasis and allostatic load. *Annals of the New York Academy of Sciences, 840*, 33--44. https://doi.org/10.1111/j.1749-6632.1998.tb09546.x

McKenna, K. M., Hashimoto, D. A., Maguire, M. S., & Bynum, W. E. (2016). The missing link: Connection is the key to resilience in medical education. *Academic Medicine, 91*(9), 1197--1199. https://doi.org/10.1097/ACM.0000000000001311

Mills, L. M., Stenfors, T., Duffy, M., Young, J. Q., Boscardin, C., ten Cate, O., & O'Sullivan, P. S. (2024). "When you're in it, it feels like it's everything": Medical students' experience of failure and remediation in the United States and the

Netherlands. *Academic Medicine, 99*(11), 1254--1259. https://doi.org/10.1097/ACM.0000000000005845

Monrouxe, L. V. (2010). Identity, identification and medical education: Why should we care? *Medical Education, 44*(1), 40--49. https://doi.org/10.1111/j.1365-2923.2009.03440.x

Montreuil, J., Lacasse, M., Audétat, M.-C., Boileau, É., Laferrière, M.-C., Lafleur, A., & Steinert, Y. (2025). Interventions for undergraduate and postgraduate medical learners with academic difficulties: A BEME systematic review update: BEME Guide No. 85. *Medical Teacher*. Advance online publication. https://doi.org/10.1080/0142159X.2024.2331041

Neff, K. D. (2003). Self-compassion: An alternative conceptualization of a healthy attitude toward oneself. *Self and Identity, 2*(2), 85--101. https://doi.org/10.1080/15298860309032

Percival, C. S., Wyatt, T. R., Martin, P. C., & Maggio, L. A. (2026). Remediation in health professions education: A scoping review of reviews. *Academic Medicine, 101*(7), 858--868. https://doi.org/10.1093/acamed/wvag003

Sawatsky, A. P., Monrouxe, L. V., Matchett, C. L., Varpio, L., Teunissen, P. W., & Usher, E. L. (2026). Professional identity struggles in healthcare professions education: A theoretical review. *Medical Education.* Advance online publication. https://doi.org/10.1111/medu.70235

Sirois, F. M., & Pychyl, T. A. (2013). Procrastination and the priority of short-term mood regulation: Consequences for future self. *Social and Personality Psychology Compass, 7*(2), 115--127. https://doi.org/10.1111/spc3.12011

Tangney, J. P., & Dearing, R. L. (2002). *Shame and guilt.* Guilford Press.

ten Cate, O., Gruppen, L. D., Kogan, J. R., Lingard, L. A., & Teunissen, P. W. (2018). Time-variable training in medicine: Theoretical considerations. *Academic Medicine, 93*(3S), S6--S11. https://doi.org/10.1097/ACM.0000000000002065

Watkins, E. R. (2008). Constructive and unconstructive repetitive thought. *Psychological Bulletin, 134*(2), 163--206. https://doi.org/10.1037/0033-2909.134.2.163

Watling, C. (2014). Cognition, culture, and credibility: Deconstructing feedback in medical education. *Perspectives on Medical Education, 3*(2), 124--128. https://doi.org/10.1007/s40037-014-0115-2

Watling, C., Driessen, E., van der Vleuten, C. P. M., Vanstone, M., & Lingard, L. (2012). Learning from clinical work: The roles of learning cues and credibility judgements. *Medical Education, 46*(2), 192--200. https://doi.org/10.1111/j.1365-2923.2011.04126.x

Worden, J. W. (2009). *Grief counseling and grief therapy: A handbook for the mental health practitioner* (4th ed.). Springer Publishing Company.

Notes for Educators and Supervisors

This section gathers guidance for educators and supervisors from across the book. Each entry can be read on its own or alongside the chapter it references.

On Chapter 1: Setbacks Are Part of the Training Landscape

Clear information gives a learner a better chance of responding effectively. Describe what happened, what standard was not met, what consequence follows, and what still needs to be clarified. Terms such as *weak*, *concerning*, or *unprofessional* are difficult to use unless they are connected to observable behavior. Specific feedback does not lower expectations or remove responsibility. It gives the learner a problem they can actually address.

On Chapter 2: The Event Is Not the Whole Story

Feedback is easier to use when it remains attached to observable behavior. Describe what happened, identify the expected standard, explain the consequence, and clarify what information is still needed. A statement such as *your assessment and plan did not consistently prioritize the most likely diagnoses* gives the learner a starting point. A statement such as *you lack clinical judgment* asks the learner to interpret a much broader judgment with much less information. Specific feedback makes both improvement and fair evaluation easier.

On Chapter 3: Why Thinking Gets Harder After a Setback

A learner who appears disorganized or slow to respond may need closer assessment before the behavior is interpreted. Avoidance, confusion, missing information, unclear expectations, cognitive overload, and genuine lack of follow-through can look similar from the outside. Some learners may also be dealing with a health problem or level of distress that requires appropriate clinical support. Reducing ambiguity does not lower expectations for timely action. It makes it easier to identify what is preventing the learner from meeting them.

On Chapter 7: Avoidance Makes Sense and Still Has a Cost

A learner who appears avoidant may need more than a reminder to follow through. Clarify the task, the deadline, and what successful completion actually requires, then find out what is preventing engagement. The barrier may be fear, confusion, missing information, poor organization, inadequate capacity, or a condition in the learning environment that needs attention. Some of those problems require accountability, while others require clarification or structural change. Understanding the function of the avoidance makes the response more precise.

On Chapter 8: Accountability Without Self-Condemnation

Learners need feedback that allows them to own what is theirs without being reduced to it. Describe the behavior, the standard, the consequence, and what successful correction would look like. A learner who has made a serious mistake may need direct language and meaningful consequences. Humiliation does not make those consequences more educational. Specific accountability gives the learner a clearer path toward demonstrating change.

On Chapter 10: Recovery Has Infrastructure

A technically sound remediation plan can fail when the surrounding conditions make it impossible to execute. Ask whether the learner has protected time, appropriate supervision, clear expectations, and realistic logistical conditions for the work being assigned. If those conditions are missing, adding more requirements may create the appearance of rigor without improving learning. Learner responsibility still matters, but the institution also owns the conditions it controls. A plan should test competence rather than endurance of an impossible system.

On Chapter 11: Recovery Is Relational

Learners may hesitate to seek help because the same institution offering support also controls progression. That tension should be acknowledged directly, especially when confidentiality has limits. Be clear about your role, what information you can keep private, and what decisions you can or cannot make. A learner is more likely to use support well when the function of the relationship is explicit. Trust grows more easily when expectations are clear.

On Chapter 12: The Setback May Have Taken Something

Learners may be dealing with more than the formal consequence written in the remediation plan. Cohort separation, financial cost, changed geography, disrupted relationships, or loss of an expected career path may shape how the learner experiences the event. Those consequences should not be assumed, because the same event may carry very different meaning for different people. Ask what changed instead of deciding what the learner must be grieving. Clear recognition of loss does not require turning the event into a therapeutic process.

On Chapter 13: The Timeline Changed. What Does That Mean?

Timeline changes can carry consequences that extend well beyond the formal academic decision. A learner repeating a year may be managing financial strain, cohort separation, visa concerns, or changes in family and career plans. Those effects should not be assumed, but they should be possible to discuss. Educators can help by separating the reason for the delay, the requirements for future progression, and the consequences that follow from the additional time. Clear standards make it less likely that chronology itself becomes a permanent label.

On Chapter 14: Returning to the Room

A learner who has completed remediation needs more than permission to return. They need clear criteria for what successful reintegration looks like and confidence that new evidence can change how they are assessed. Increased observation may be appropriate, but it should have a defined purpose and endpoint. Programs should distinguish necessary monitoring from indefinite suspicion. **A developmental process should contain a credible way to move beyond the label.**

On Chapter 15: What Story Will This Become?

Educators can unintentionally encourage learners to build overly large stories around setbacks. Questions such as *What did this teach you about yourself?* or *How did this make you stronger?* may push meaning before the learner has enough distance or evidence to answer. A more useful approach is to ask what happened, what changed, and what the learner understands differently now. That leaves room for growth, loss, ambiguity, or very little lasting meaning. Reflection should improve accuracy rather than force redemption.

On Chapter 16: Recovery Is Part of Professional Formation

Professional formation should leave room for correction, changed direction, and updated evidence. Learners need to know that a mistake or remediation process can be taken seriously without becoming a permanent identity assignment. Institutions should also examine what they were responsible for changing when supervision, workload, policy, or learning conditions contributed to the problem. Development requires the possibility that both learner and environment can respond to new evidence. A system that demands growth from the learner while refusing to revise itself applies professional formation in only one direction.

www.ingramcontent.com/pod-product-compliance
Lightning Source LLC
LaVergne TN
LVHW030726061126
851857LV00019B/2017
9798997892807